A Namaste Care Activity Book

Sensory Stories and Activities for People Living with Advanced Dementia

NICOLA KENDALL

With chapters from Emma Biglands, Paul Chazot, Lourdes Colclough, Laura Johnston, Michelle Kindleysides, Andrea Lambell, Richard Langdon, Colette O'Driscoll, Magda Pasak and Susannah Thwaites

Foreword by Rishi Jawaheer – Director of Namaste Care International

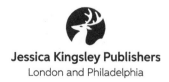

Jessica Kingsley Publishers
London and Philadelphia

First published in Great Britain in 2021 by Jessica Kingsley Publishers
An Hachette Company

1

Copyright © Nicola Kendall 2021
Chapters 4, 6, 7, 8, 9, 10 and 11 copyright © Jessica Kingsley Publishers 2021
Foreword copyright © Rishi Jawaheer 2021

Box 6.2 reproduced and adapted with kind permission of Abscent.

Front cover image source: Shutterstock®.

A CIP catalogue record for this title is available from the
British Library and the Library of Congress

ISBN 978 1 78775 493 5
eISBN 978 1 78775 494 2

Printed and bound in Great Britain by CPI Group

Jessica Kingsley Publishers' policy is to use papers that are natural, renewable and recyclable
products and made from wood grown in sustainable forests. The logging and manufacturing
processes are expected to conform to the environmental regulations of the country of origin.

Jessica Kingsley Publishers
Carmelite House
50 Victoria Embankment
London EC4Y 0DZ

www.jkp.com

*In memory of all our Namaste Care friends
that we have loved and lost.*

Contents

Section 3: Sensory Stories and Activities

What I would say if I could…

Please don't say that I'm already gone. It might seem that way, but I'm here, honestly, I am. It's just that I can't communicate the way I used to anymore. Even after I die, I won't be gone. I exist in the memory of those who know and love me. Don't give up on me. Enter my world. It's a world of sensations and basic needs. Simple pleasures mean a lot to me now. Please believe that love, attention and care are more powerful than my dementia. Don't be afraid. Come and find me.

I'm still here.

Foreword

Rishi Jawaheer – Director of Namaste Care International

Growing up in a dementia care home, where my sister and I shared a single room at the top of our house, Homelands, with our parents Roy and Sherine, we saw the 14 residents as members of our extended family. Having begun their careers as registered mental health nurses, both our parents already had many years' experience of running day hospitals in the NHS. Since those early beginnings at Homelands, their dedication to providing person-centred specialist dementia care has seen the Jawa Group grow into one of London's leading care villages. This family-centric ethos inspired me to join the company and I have gone on to lead the Jawa Group.

When we first met Professor Joyce Simard and Min Stacpoole, we recognized them as kindred spirits. Namaste Care gave a name to what we had always believed in – 'honouring the spirit within'. It sparked something within us, and we came to embrace Namaste Care wholeheartedly in our care homes. Not only did we foster our connection with the intervention's pioneers, we also wanted to help promote it to like-minded individuals.

In collaboration with Joyce, Min and Namaste Care practitioners around the world, in September 2018, Namaste Care International was launched at an inaugural conference at the premises of the Jawa Group. Gillian Hensley-Gray from our team has played a pivotal role in supporting the expansion of Namaste Care and has been by my side. Nicola Kendall was one of the first delegates through the door, and with a shared passion for the quiet revolution that is Namaste Care, we have got to know Nicola well, not only as a colleague but also as a friend. Her approach to adapting namaste to real life situations and context makes things accessible and relevant to people in care. We have seen first-hand how her approach can transform the wellbeing and outlook of all involved. This also gives the carers another outlet of expression and brings variety and energy to the dedicated work they do. This is very much at the heart of what we do and this has always been at the forefront of my agenda to change the negative perception of care and encourage the next generation of carers to come through. Namaste Care and Champions like Nicola set the tone for valuing carers and challenging society not to stick to stereotypes, and put carers on the pedestal in society that is often reserved for the traditional roles of doctors and lawyers. Carers make the world go round!

Now Nicola is Namaste Care International's Champion for Hospices, one of 17 Champions worldwide. Her initiative at St Cuthbert's Hospice in Durham, to 'take the hospice to the community', supports people with advanced dementia to stay at home for longer.

In this time of pandemic, Namaste Care has more relevance than ever to those in care homes, hospices and hospitals. The positive effects on people with advanced illness, and their families, can be seen every day in care settings of all shapes and sizes.

Nicola's book will give Namaste Care practitioners all the creative tools they need to deliver the loving touch and meaningful activity that is central to this way of life, which can bring so much joy and comfort to those who have been alone for so long.

Rishi Jawaheer
The Jawa Group, London
Namaste Care International
Care Vision CMS

INTRODUCTION

How do we live, rather than just exist?

That's a question we should all ask ourselves, whether we have dementia or not, isn't it?

When it comes to the advanced stages of dementia, however, that question becomes even more urgent and powerful. In the last few years and months of our lives, how do we want to live?

Victor Frankl put it thus:

> We must never forget that we may find meaning in life even when confronted with a hopeless situation, when facing a fate that cannot be changed. For what then matters is to bear witness to the uniquely human potential at its best, which is to transform a personal tragedy into a triumph, to turn one's predicament into a human achievement. (Frankl 2004, p.116)

Every time I look into the eyes of someone living with advanced dementia, I see a light in their eyes which dementia has not dimmed. They are still there, they haven't been lost, even though it can feel like they have.

If you are reading this book, then you already care about helping someone living with advanced dementia to live with quality in their lives, rather than to just exist. I don't need to convince you of the why; you are interested in the how. Namaste Care offers the opportunity to LIVE, with meaning, joy and connection right up to the moment we take our last breath, by offering simple, sensory experiences within a safe and relaxed space. Namaste Care, at its very core, facilitates a special form of genuine close attention between two people, and allows for an appropriate giving and receiving of love.

The idea for this book came about following a review I carried out with a family who had a volunteer Namaste Care visitor. The family was very grateful for the time the volunteer was giving, but they were concerned that the volunteer was tentative about trying out sensory activities. I had to reflect on my abilities as a trainer and project supervisor to be fair, but I also realized that not everyone is creative and imaginative when it comes to thinking of sensory activities. So, this book began to take shape and evolve in my mind into what it is now: a resource book of themed activities linked to sensory stories to inspire and guide a themed Namaste Care session.

Joyce Simard, who developed Namaste Care in the USA, encourages us to think about that central question: How do we live, rather than just exist, with quality and meaning in our lives? I hope this book contributes to the growing interest in Namaste Care as an answer to this question.

Section 1, 'Inspiring Creativity in Namaste Care', provides a foundation for the rest of the book. It summarizes the Namaste Care approach and the need for sensory stimulation, which is covered in more detail in my book *Namaste Care for People Living with Advanced Dementia: A Practical Guide for Carers and Professionals* (Kendall 2019). I also discuss sensory storytelling and give guidance about how to tell a sensory story. This supports the core purpose of the book, which is encouraging the use of the sensory stories and associated activities found in Section 3. Section 1 additionally includes a contribution from Colette O'Driscoll from St Joseph's Hospice in Hackney, London, and Lourdes Colclough from Macmillan, which discusses respecting cultural diversity in Namaste Care. This section concludes with some guidance about helping a person to live, right up until they take their last breath, with consideration about end of life support.

Section 2, 'Supporting Sensory Approaches', contains guidance and discussions from a variety of very knowledgeable professionals, aimed at further supporting a sensory approach and focusing on the various senses, one at a time. I am incredibly grateful to each contributor for generously sharing their expertise and experience.

Andrea Lambell starts this section by giving us detailed advice in Chapter 6 about the use of aromatherapy. It is a powerful tool for wellbeing when used safely. You may not have ever thought about taking the person living with dementia to an aromatherapist or having this type of treatment, but this is an option that is worth exploring given the growing evidence about its benefits.

In Chapter 7 Paul Chazot and Laura Johnston from Durham University then discuss the therapeutic use of lighting and how this can be used to improve orientation and wellbeing by telling us about the 'Enlighten Project'. Again, the idea is to get us thinking about how we can use these ideas in a home or care setting.

We next take a 'trip down memory lane' via our tastebuds in Chapter 8, as Michelle Kindlysides from Beamish Museum explores the pleasurable associations of food and memory.

In Chapter 9, Susannah Thwaites and Emma Biglands (occupational therapists championing the use of Namaste Care in Tees, Esk and Wear Valley

NHS Trust) focus on using the sense of touch to connect and all the issues that relate to this, such as consent.

One of our own Namaste Care volunteers from St Cuthbert's Hospice, Richard Langdon, reflects on his experience of using music as a powerful way to build a bond with the fabulous Cyril in Chapter 10. Hearing a volunteer's experience and how it has touched him in the way that it has, is completely heart-warming and reflects how rewarding it is to offer someone the Namaste Care approach.

Finally, in Chapter 11, Magda Pasak from St Cuthbert's offers a physiotherapy perspective on the importance of encouraging activity and movement for as long as possible to promote wellbeing.

Section 3 contains a selection of themed stories with ideas for sensory activities that would support and enhance each story. This section is designed to be dipped into and to match to the interests and experiences of people living with dementia. I would love for people to be inspired to write and use their own stories, as these can be much more personalized and specific to the person.

A word, here, about cultural neutrality. As I began to write some sensory stories, it became very obvious how deeply embedded our own cultural history and biases are. I began to write stories that were very much steeped in the traditions of the North East of England, which is my home. I realized I needed to make stories as culturally neutral as possible, to make them more widely relevant across regions, countries and cultures, but I know I will have failed in eliminating my own history, interests and preferences. I would therefore encourage you to write your own culture-specific sensory stories, once you get the idea, and these stories can be tailored to the life history and beliefs of the person living with dementia.

I have also tried to give some thought to what might misdirect or confuse a person living with dementia. For example, I planned to write a story about going on holiday but I realized this could prompt people to think they were indeed going on holiday. Instead I have tried to create stories which evoke a mood or capture the feel of a moment. You could equally write a sensory story about a real-life event or a fiction story. I have kept the stories as neutral as I can and I hope you can personalize them more with the sensory objects and experiences you choose to offer along with them.

My aim in writing this book, therefore, is to create inspiration and ideas, which may well lead to you developing your own unique themes and sensory stories that are matched to the person you are supporting, as you know them best. I hope this book is concise and accessible enough to allow you to dip in. I advise our Namaste Care volunteers to approach each session with gentle curiosity, a relaxed shrug of the shoulders and an attitude of 'let's just try it and see what happens', and so I would urge you to do the same.

Happy exploring…

REFERENCES

Frankl, V. (2004) *Man's Search for Meaning*. London: Ebury. First published in German in 1946 under the title *Ein Psycholog erlebt das Konzentrationslager*.

Kendall, N. (2019) *Namaste Care for People Living with Advanced Dementia: A Practical Guide for Carers and Professionals*. London: Jessica Kingsley Publishers.

INSPIRING CREATIVITY IN NAMASTE CARE

1

NAMASTE CARE

Namaste Care is a gentle, sensory approach aimed at 'honouring the spirit within'. It is incredibly hard to do it justice with any verbal or written description, as what happens between two people in a Namaste Care session is beyond words. I will nevertheless attempt to capture the essence of it by sharing some thoughts and experiences in this chapter.

NB. A full description of Namaste Care is available in Joyce Simard's book, *The End of Life Namaste Care Programme for People with Dementia* (Simard 2013), or my book, *Namaste Care for People Living with Advanced Dementia: A Practical Guide for Carers and Professionals* (Kendall 2019).

What I believe makes the person receiving Namaste Care feel so special is that during the time you spend with them *they are the centre of your universe*. You are entirely interested in and focused on them and being with them. The more I experience sharing Namaste Care, the more I realize that the core conditions necessary for a session are the same as for a psychological therapy session; that is:

- a safe space
- being genuine and curious
- showing unconditional positive regard
- giving focused attention
- use of empathy
- free from distractions
- acceptance
- patience
- non-judgement
- a gentle pace
- expressing love.

If we were ethically able to measure hormone levels before and after a Namaste Care session, I am convinced that we would see a reduction in the stress hormones cortisol and adrenaline and an increase in the feel-good, wellbeing hormones serotonin and oxytocin. There's a PhD study in that for someone, surely? I may have to explore that idea further myself!

Psychotherapist Dr Sue Gerhardt explains the effects of hormones in our bodies:

> Every day of our lives, our internal biochemicals are fluctuating outside our awareness. All sorts of emotional and physiological responses are taking place automatically. Waves of hormones come and go through the day, adjusting and responding to events outside the body, or inside the body. They are involved in the daily rhythms of sleeping and waking, processing food, and keeping warm, mostly under the influence of the hypothalamus in the core limbic area of the brain. These chemicals set off gene expression, changing behaviour in a way that will hopefully help the organism to maintain a good state. (Gerhardt 2004, p.58)

The internal regulation achieved by the hypothalamus can be damaged by some types of dementia, affecting sleep, awareness of hunger, temperature regulation, behaviour and many other things, so it is difficult to be absolutely sure without scientific research whether Namaste Care can generate these feel-good hormones. However, we consistently observe improved mood, a reduction in pain, increased eye contact, reaching out for human touch, smiles and laughter, which would point to improved wellbeing and a consistently positive effect. Namaste Care does not really have any contraindications, other than the person living with dementia indicating to us that they don't want the interaction.

If we summarize the types of activities that promote 'feel-good hormones', Namaste Care covers a lot of them.

Oxytocin – the 'love' hormone	Serotonin – mood balancing
Playing with a dog or cat	Exercise
Hugging	A walk/being outside in nature
Human touch/hand holding	Meditation
Giving a compliment	Music
Holding, cuddling and playing with a baby	Sunshine
Endorphins – pain relieving	Dopamine – sense of reward
Laughter	Eating food
Essential oils	Completing a task
Exercise	Self-care activities/being pampered
Dark chocolate	Celebrating achievements

It is difficult to provide an exact template for a Namaste Care session, as it will vary depending on whether it is a group or one-to-one situation, what the needs of the people receiving Namaste Care are and what we know about their life stories. The following is a brief summary of what could normally be included in a Namaste Care session:

- a pre-prepared and homely environment
- a warm and personal greeting
- a check on the person's pain levels and mood
- moving them to a comfortable chair
- tucking them up with a warm, cosy blanket
- soothing music playing, favourite music of the person, or music matched to the sensory theme
- use of a room spritz or diffuser
- natural objects in the room, such as flowers
- encouraging the person to take frequent drinks
- focused one-to-one attention (in a group, this would mean spending one-to-one time with one person then moving on)
- washing hands, face, feet
- hair brushing
- a hand massage, foot massage, scalp massage
- applying face cream
- gentle passive movements to joints
- honouring the seasons
- looking at pictures in books or photo albums appropriate to the person's interests
- exploring tactile objects
- realistic animals and dolls
- reading to the person
- sharing a snack that the person would consider a treat.

Joyce Simard developed Namaste Care in the USA to meet the sensory needs of people living with advanced dementia, and it was originally intended as a small group activity for care home residents. It is proving to be entirely transferable into a range of environments, however, and has spread to be used in numerous countries around the world, including Australia, Greece, the Netherlands, the Czech Republic and Iceland.

Through my project based at St Cuthbert's Hospice in Durham, UK, we deliver Namaste Care sessions to people in their own home, we visit people who have dementia on a care of the elderly ward in an acute hospital, we have developed a Namaste Care-inspired garden group and have recently introduced it into our hospice inpatient unit for anyone receiving care.

This last initiative is proving especially exciting because it means that people with conditions other than dementia are having the Namaste Care experience. Whereas it is difficult to gain feedback from a person living with advanced dementia, other than by observation or carer comments, someone who has cancer can give us clear feedback. What they are telling us is that they have less pain by the end of a session and that they feel more relaxed and content.

A Namaste Care visit, whether it is in hospital, a hospice, a care home or other setting, allows the professionals or family carers involved to really slow down and take time to truly be with someone and to share nurturing activities that are not merely task-driven. The benefit is undoubtedly a two-way thing. Our volunteers regularly tell me that they gain as much from sharing this time as does the person they are visiting, and research carried out by St Christopher's Hospice in London showed that Namaste Care sessions improved staff morale.

With a growing understanding that care homes are becoming hospices as the common place of death for people living with dementia, a general drive to improve end of life care is gaining momentum, and Namaste Care can be very much a part of that. George Coxon, an owner of two care homes in South West England, reflects:

> As the former end of life lead commissioner for Devon and concurrent care home owner, the manner that I approach end of life care has both front line exposure and strategic aspects of 'what we said and what we did' in this area in our plan to take on the Namaste Care model – quoting often that end of life care is the most important part of care to get right.
>
> Our Namaste journey in my two small but well-regarded homely care homes in South Devon began with a chance reading of an article in a non-care related magazine, *The Economist*-sponsored *Intelligent Life* (Jan/Feb 2016), where Professor Jo Hockley (now a much-admired colleague, whom I have spent time with both formally as well as sharing pizza with in Edinburgh) wrote on the subject in an article titled 'How to have a Good Death' (based on Witham and Hockley 2016). It has so often now been cited by me in many circles and with many care home and NHS colleagues, friends and residents and loved ones in our care, too.
>
> So, to our journey, as it is a journey, and like all the best journeys of reflection, growth, change, we are not at a destination just yet. The story so far looks like this.

Preparation and immersion

There are principles that I carry with me from my many years of mental health nursing and the time spent reading and absorbing ideas of different therapy models and constructs. All have led me to now describing myself as an eclecticist or integrationist in my approach to care frameworks, meaning someone who draws on a wide spectrum of models of care. Reading about Namaste Care for those living and dying with advanced dementia has meant for me a process of reaching a point of readiness to commit to the approach, yet also to recognize our journey and Namaste plan is an evolving one.

The what and the how

Winning over the hearts and minds of the sceptical audience of care home staff who are often deeply suspicious of externally sourced wisdom, so regularly imported from afar, is a first hurdle that must be overcome. I will not pretend that our staff greeted my latest fantastically innovative, transformational way to look after our residents as they approach their final period of life entirely enthusiastically. We are and always were good at end of life care. CQC [Care Quality Commission] have acknowledged this in our outstanding inspection ratings, and families have testified to this too – we have personalized the kindest and most committed care imaginable, and I knew this at the point of beginning our immersion in the Namaste approach. But our care model did lack much of the person-centred ingredients enshrined in Namaste Care and we also lacked an evidence base to wrap around and embed our skills, knowledge and ways to explain to the uninitiated – the person we were caring for and their families needing reassurance and clarity of what lay ahead.

After attending one of Professor Hockley's workshops in September 2019, having been invited to Edinburgh to share the work we are doing in Devon, I returned south, fully inspired and ready to embark upon our local plan.

Firstly, I spoke with both our home managers, setting out the vision and implementation plan we would be taking forward. This involved leading some informal introductory sessions using Nicola Kendall's book *Namaste Care for People Living with Advanced Dementia*, combined with the *Toolkit for Implementing the Namaste programme* from St Christopher's Hospice (Stacpoole, Thompsell and Hockley 2016). Although there is so much more to read, I was and am determined to maintain a view that too much reading can limit a plan and slow progress – I will defend strongly the view of having perhaps 2–3 central guides and integrating a plan in your personal setting or context and developing and learning as you go. I presented our work and plan at the November 2019 HospiceUK annual conference in Liverpool to a very discerning and expert audience of mostly palliative care specialists, where I described what we were doing in adapting and applying the Namaste Care approach.

My trip to Liverpool also afforded me the opportunity to visit a fellow outstanding-rated care home in Warwickshire who have fully embraced

Namaste Care and in a most impressive way. Galanos House, a large British Legion home, has become one of my four primary influencers regarding our approach, the others being Nicola Kendall, Jo Hockley and Isabelle Latham (an academic with a special interest in Namaste Care at Worcester University). I am connected with Isabelle via a research project supported by the Alzheimer's Society.

Ongoing learning

Although we are early in our journey, we are well underway in our progress. We have appointed three Namaste Champions, provided enhanced training, offered an enhanced pay for the role and commenced our implementation with the few residents we have looked after at the end of their lives. I too have been part of the care, using the guide and recommended specific care recommendations so unique to Namaste.

I have led workshops in my recent role as Network Associate at the South West Academic Health and Science Network (SW AHSN) for fellow care home activists keen to develop their own implementation plan and also for SW AHSN staff interested in the approach.

Ongoing learning means being reflective about our own approach – aspiring to do better and be better as well as being receptive to others and always open to improvement. When we hold our regular staff briefings, residents and guests meetings and in-house training, quality huddles, staff 1:1s and pep talks, we often use a simple self-scoring system of 1–10, low to high, in sharing how well we are doing. Staff never score themselves a 10 and we all agree there is always more to learn and ways to make changes – our care plans are person-centred and our Namaste Care is always seen as essential co-production between the person, their loved ones and ourselves – we have shared the model with families and also promoted the essential principle of the Namaste Care partnership being so vital.

The journey continues and the learning too. This second book by Nicola will add yet more ways to inspire others to join this end of life care revolution, as we did only a year ago – many more will follow if I have my way, too.

George Coxon is a leader in the field of residential care, demanding high-quality care for his residents, and he is widely recognized for his inspiring and excellent work. He is a real example of the difference that placing heart and soul into your work and genuine, loving (and fun) care can make to the lives of individuals. I am not surprised that Namaste Care struck a chord with him. It does to those with the heart for it.

BEGINNING TO EXPLORE WHY NAMASTE CARE WORKS

If we think about the key elements of Namaste Care, we can try to match each to their function. We know that they work from experience and observations, but this table shows why I think they work. This area requires a lot more research, and so the following table is based on my *opinion and observations*. It's essentially a hypothesis I need to find ways to test.

Core element of Namaste Care	Function
A pre-prepared and homely environment	Decreases the possibility of distractions and welcomes the person into a calm, relaxing space. Allows the carer to be centred and prepared for the session.
A warm and personal greeting	Person-centred, acknowledging who the person is, respecting their preferences and gaining their attention.
A check on the person's pain levels and mood	Allows us to address any pain issues before starting a session, and also gives us a steer about what approach may be needed in the session (uplifting, relaxing, calming or energetic).
Moving them to a comfortable chair	Wheelchairs do not provide adequate seating due to lack of support. A comfortable chair, ideally a recliner, will allow the person to feel fully supported and able to relax.
Tucking them up with a warm, cosy blanket	Provides lots of sensory feedback to help the person's sense of their body in space (proprioception) and thus to feel more secure and safe. It may also evoke pleasant memories from childhood about being 'tucked in' for bed.
Soothing music playing, favourite music of the person, or music matched to the sensory theme	Stimulates across the whole brain, evoking memories and influencing mood. Allows us to personalize care by choosing the person's favourite music. Is a universal means of reaching and connecting with people.
Use of a room spritz or diffuser	Can affect mood and memory through smell receptors being directly wired to memory in the brain.
Encouraging the person to take frequent drinks	Increasing hydration levels will reduce the possibility of urine and chest infections, as well as improving cognition, keeping the skin hydrated and aiding general comfort.
Focused one-to-one attention	Boosts a sense of wellbeing and self-worth. Gives a very strong message that the person with dementia is important and interesting. Enables the person with dementia to focus, usually intently on our face, and to 'be with' us in a very genuine way.

cont.

Core element of Namaste Care	Function
Washing hands, face, feet	A very functional task which can be carried out in a much slower, more meaningful and sensory way during a Namaste Care session.
Hair brushing	A very soothing, relational and personal activity that people find relaxing and may remind them of being cared for as a child.
A hand massage, foot massage, scalp massage	Providing a soothing connection through gentle human touch. Very relaxing and loving. Helps to soothe joints, calms breathing and improves skin integrity.
Applying face cream	Soothing and pleasant experience which also promotes skin comfort and moisture levels at a time when skin can become fragile and dry.
Gentle passive movements to joints	As people lose their mobility, joints and muscles become stiff and painful. Encouraging movement, even if as the carer we have to support that movement, will help keep joints and muscles as mobile as possible, given that these symptoms will inevitably progress.
Honouring the seasons	Helping with the person in making sense of the world and orientating them to the weather, the season and a sense of place and time.
Looking at pictures in books or photo albums	Stimulating vision with interesting or familiar places and people can be good at engaging and holding the person's interest.
Exploring tactile objects	The person with dementia will lose their fine motor skills as their symptoms progress, but they are still able to explore the world through touch until towards the very end of their life.
Realistic animals and dolls	These enable the person to express their instinctive nurturing abilities and feel comforted.
Reading to the person	The soothing and relational sound of a human voice. May evoke memories of bedtime stories and family time. Especially nice if the person always enjoyed reading but is no longer able to concentrate to read for themselves.
Sharing a snack that the person would consider a treat	Pleasant memories and the pleasure of eating something we enjoy. Increased dopamine levels from the idea that this is a 'naughty treat'.

From years of delivering Namaste Care, I *know* that it works, and is something that both professionals and carers crave, which is a more meaningful way to support someone who may seem to have already been lost but is very much still there, waiting for us to connect with them in a way that now makes sense to them. I hope this book provides the inspiration and confidence to give it a try.

REFERENCES

Gerhardt, S. (2004) *Why Love Matters: How Affection Shapes a Baby's Brain*. Abingdon: Routledge.

Kendall, N. (2019) *Namaste Care for People Living with Advanced Dementia: A Practical Guide for Carers. and Professionals*. London: Jessica Kingsley Publishers.

Simard, J. (2013) *The End of Life Namaste Care Programme for People with Dementia*. Baltimore, MD: Health Professions Press.

Stacpoole, M., Thompsell, A. and Hockley, J. (2016) *Toolkit for Implementing the Namaste Care Programme for People with Advanced Dementia Living in Care Homes*. Available at www.stchristophers.org.uk/wp-content/uploads/2016/03/Namaste-Care-Programme-Toolkit-06.04.2016.pdf, accessed on 2 December 2020.

Witham, M.D. and Hockley, J. (2016) 'A good death for the oldest old.' *Age and Ageing 45*(3), 329–331.

2

SENSORY STIMULATION

Sensory stimulation therapy was originally developed to help the cognitive development of people with learning disabilities and autism. For people living with dementia, we can think of it more as maintenance of function, in an illness which is progressive and irreversible. It becomes, in the case of someone living with advanced dementia, a therapeutic and gentle means to communicate and make sense of a jumbled, stressful world.

Alzheimer's.net, a US online community providing advocacy, education and support for people whose lives are affected by dementia, describes sensory stimulation as using 'everyday objects to arouse one or more of the five senses (hearing, sight, smell, taste and touch) with the goal of evoking positive feelings' (Wegerer 2017). Sensory stimulation, especially for someone living with dementia, works best using familiar objects and by stimulating one sense at a time.

Good sensory items would include:

- natural objects with interesting textures, smells or colours
- favourite foods and drinks
- items that the person would recognize from their past
- a playlist of music that is meaningful to the person
- scents associated with happy memories or people
- everyday items such as a hairbrush, flannel, textured blankets
- beautifully scented massage oils and waxes
- twiddle mitts, activity boards and stress balls
- mood lamps
- aromatherapy diffusers.

Benefits of sensory stimulation can include:

- helping to preserve cognition for as long as possible
- improving concentration and alertness

- improving mental wellbeing
- helping a person to connect with memories
- providing interactive and engaging activities
- connecting a person living with dementia to other people and their surroundings
- helping to orientate and settle the person.

In 2020, we introduced Namaste Care into our inpatient unit at St Cuthbert's Hospice, Durham. For equity, we decided to offer Namaste Care to anyone receiving inpatient care, whether or not they had dementia. As mentioned in Chapter 1, this led to some interesting feedback from patients who were able to tell us how Namaste Care felt, in a way that people living with advanced dementia were not able to. However, what they told us must apply equally to the people living with dementia:

- Their pain was reduced.
- They felt happier by the end of the session.
- It broke up the loneliness of long days in one room.
- It helped them to share their memories and stories about their life, which felt very meaningful as they approached the end of their life.
- It changed the emphasis from good medical care to good holistic care.
- It helped them to feel relaxed.

In Namaste Care with people living with advanced dementia, everyday care tasks can be turned into pleasant experiences with some thought to make them sensory. For instance, washing someone's face with a face cloth scented with rose water, or helping them to wash their hands in a bowl of water that is scented with a citrusy handwash, will be an opportunity to turn an ordinary chore into an enjoyable experience.

The key always with sensory stimulation is *simplicity* and a *slow pace*. This allows the person living with dementia time to process information at their speed, not ours, and takes the pressure off them to somehow perform or 'get it right'. We are moving from 'doing to' to 'doing with'. We offer the sensory experience without expectation, watching always for signs that the person does not want to engage or does not *consent* to the interaction. These signs will most likely be non-verbal, such as a frown or pushing away something that is offered, but they are usually clear and we must always respect the wishes of the person making this choice.

In the sensory stories presented in Section 3, each story is accompanied by a list of suggested sensory resources. Choosing an appropriate story may be in response to the weather or season, or it could be in response to what you know about a person's life. For example, if the person living with dementia loved trips to the seaside, you might choose 'By the Sea'; or if the person is a fan of poetry, you could choose 'Poet's Corner'. If you are able to personalize the suggested resources based on what you know about the person, that will clearly add meaning, pleasure and comforting familiarity. In 'A Tropical Evening', for instance, my cocktail of choice would be a Long Island iced tea! For 'Mountain Stream' I picture Snowdonia in Wales, whereas someone else might think of the Alps or the Rockies. This demonstrates the importance of gathering good, sensory life story information.

Knowledge about the person's background is especially important in order to eliminate, where we can, any possible distressing stimuli. Smells and sounds especially can trigger a traumatic memory, so we need to be cautious and check for anything that the family thinks might be relevant here. If the smell of a particular brand of aftershave reminds someone of their abusive father, we would obviously never introduce that as one of their sensory stimuli. On the other hand, if the smell of lily of the valley perfume reminds someone of their mother, whom they were very close to, this would be a positive smell to share with them. We can't always have this information, but we should try to find out as much as we can.

In my book, *Namaste Care for People Living with Advanced Dementia* (Kendall 2019), I used the analogy of our brain being like a forest of neural pathways, and sensory stimulation being one way to maintain and tend the pathways as best we can. Joanna Grace (2018) also uses this metaphor and advises one strong, clear message (i.e., one stimulus at a time) to reach the other side of the forest. Another analogy might be neural pathways as the lanes of a motorway and a car being one message being sent along that lane. If the motorway is clogged up with cars, it will lead to a traffic jam. It is hard to pick out one car in a sea of cars and lorries. The person living with dementia, if overwhelmed with information, will tend either to shut down, or become frustrated and angry. Instead, sending one simple, clear message (that is one car being sent along the motorway at any one time) makes that message much easier to recognize and process.

So, in concluding this section, I would encourage you to play and have fun, while keeping sensory activities age-appropriate and respectful. As Grace reflects:

> We may long to be able to connect and communicate with them in the ways that we did before, or in the ways that are normal to us, and not being able to do so is disheartening. When we seek instead to have sensory conversations we open up the possibility of connecting with them as they are now. (Grace 2018, p.180)

This requires us to adapt to the current reality and demands a level of acceptance from us which we may have been resisting. But in return, the responses, the smiles and laughter, the magic moments generated, are more than worth it.

REFERENCES

Grace, J. (2018) *Sharing Sensory Stories and Conversations with People with Dementia: A Practical Guide.* London: Jessica Kingsley Publishers.

Kendall, N. (2019) *Namaste Care for People Living with Advanced Dementia: A Practical Guide for Carers and Professionals.* London: Jessica Kingsley Publishers.

Wegerer, J. (2017) 'How sensory stimulation can help Alzheimer's.' Available at www.alzheimers.net/2014-01-23/sensory-stimulation-alzheimers-patients, accessed on 4 December 2020.

3

SENSORY STORYTELLING

Storytelling is as old as human communication. Before the written word, stories were how traditions, lessons and histories were passed on. This oral tradition is deeply embedded in our human experience as noted by Joe Griffin and Ivan Tyrrell: 'Stories contain the wisdom of the species, because knowledge is metaphorically expressed through them and transmitted orally down the generations' (Griffin and Tyrrell 2003, p.228).

Think of our ancient ancestors sitting around a fire and exchanging stories. Tales of giants and gods, heroes and villains, have helped to shape us and our society. Often our bedtime routine may have involved stories being read to us by a parent or grandparent to help us settle and relax before sleep. In our first few years in nursery and school there was story time. Thus, storytelling is relational and relaxing. It uses words and narrative that evoke our feelings and senses and help us to experience the world with a shared understanding. This is because stories activate the right hemisphere of our brain, which is creative and understands patterns, as opposed to the left hemisphere, which deals with facts and logic. With dementia, both hemispheres of the brain are affected, but the right side can be accessed and stimulated by creating the right atmosphere and feeling. By creating a safe and calm environment for 'story time', we stand more chance of being able to evoke pleasant memories and emotions. John and Caitlin Matthews reflect lyrically on the history of storytelling this way:

> Once upon a time... when people still lived in caves and sat around the camp fire every night, storytellers used their magic to keep the vast and silent darkness at bay. Their tales hopped off the tongue and into the ear, taking root in the imagination of their listeners. There, each story grew wide and tall, put flesh on its bones, and then walked about in the world. (Matthews and Matthews 2009, p.9)

The Namaste Care approach of being made comfortable and tucked up with a cosy blanket is an ideal preparation for a story. It will encourage feelings of safety, being cared for and loved. The story can then be used as a vehicle for sensory stimulation that is meaningful to the person and not abstract. So, let's now explore in more detail the idea of a *sensory* story.

SENSORY STORIES

Joanna Grace describes sensory stories as 'concise texts, typically less than ten sentences, in which each line of text is partnered with a richly stimulating and relevant sensory experience' (Grace 2018, p.95).

There are some key points to make about sensory stories, which although being much shorter than a standard story, are no less of a story. They are accommodating a person with dementia's changing needs and difficulties with processing larger amounts of information. Grace writes:

> All of our brains have a limited processing capacity and when we are struggling with our health, be that mental or physical, our resources are depleted. Language places huge processing demands on the brain. You will know from times when you have felt stressed or ill that you need peace and quiet, you do NOT want lots and lots of words. By reducing the number of words we use in a conversation, or whilst sharing a story, we reduce the demands placed on someone's processing capacity and thus we make it easier for them to listen to us. (Grace 2018, pp.97–98)

Taking together the guidance on sensory stories from Grace's (2018) *Sharing Sensory Stories and Conversations with People with Dementia: A Practical Guide*, as well as my own experience of sharing therapeutic stories in psychotherapy, we can begin to build a consistent approach which will support a Namaste Care sensory storytelling session.

Preparation

As with all Namaste Care sessions, preparing all the resources that you plan to use beforehand will ensure that the session flows and has minimal disruptions. Part of your preparation could include reading through the sensory story to yourself a few times to become familiar with it and plan how you will read it. You can also lay out the resources that you plan to use so that they are easily accessible as the story goes along. Check any electrical items are working properly and the environment is set up in a way that will enhance the story. Does the lighting need to be subdued or bright? Have you got everything you need to make the person comfortable, such as a reclining chair, blankets, cushions, pillows? People living with dementia do not have the cognitive ability to cope easily with muddles and disruption, so preparation time is especially important.

Gaining attention

The first line of each story is designed to grab the attention of the person you are reading to. Ensure they can see you clearly and look up at the end of the first line to make eye contact and smile. This first line should be read in an especially engaging, upbeat way.

Repetition

There is something familiar and soothing about repetition. It is a technique often used in children's stories to enhance how a child interacts with the story. A story introduced in the earlier stages of dementia and often repeated can bring relaxation and reminiscence as the dementia symptoms progress. It provides an anchor in what feels to people living with dementia like a confusing, unstable and anxiety-provoking world: 'Re-telling the sensory story as dementia progresses should maintain the familiarity and predictability of the stimuli' (Leighton, Oddy and Grace 2016, p.2).

In each session I would consider repeating the story twice. The first time is a slow read-through to introduce the theme of the session. The second time is a repeat but with all of the supporting sensory stimuli and activities added in.

Consistency

We don't live in an ideal world, and this may not be possible, but consistency in the storyteller is really helpful wherever we can manage it. This is easier to achieve with family carers than in a care home, but if it is possible to have, say, the activity co-ordinator always reading the story, with care assistants supporting, that would be ideal.

We might be tempted to add words to the story because they are so simple and minimal and we want to add to the experience. However, given that the stories are designed to account for the person's processing difficulties, it is better to read them exactly as they are. This will allow for consistency between different people reading the story and will allow the person to fully experience the sensory activities that go alongside it.

Style and pace

I would recommend reading the story slowly, clearly and deliberately, speaking each word lyrically as if you were giving the person a wondrous gift. Allow time at the end of each sentence for the person to respond and acknowledge any response they give. Processing time may vary between people, and we generally are not good with silence, so we need to breathe, be patient and wait. Grace writes:

> It can be hard to sit and hold space with a person as you wait for a response that takes minutes to come, but what a wonderful thing to be able to do: to be the person who hears a person who is normally unheard. What a precious role to play in someone's life, to be the one who waits long enough to hear them. (Grace 2018, p.105)

Knowing the person

Each sensory story in Section 3 has a list of suggested sensory experiences and resources that might accompany that story. However, you can personalize the story and any activities of objects that you use, according to what you know of the person's life history.

Responses

The kind of response we might expect is obviously going to vary widely, depending on the person, their type of dementia, what kind of day they are having, as well as many other variables. We might get a verbal 'I remember when…' response from them, or a phrase or word. We may have movement, reaching out to touch, joining in with an activity or tapping a rhythm. We may see a smile, a sigh or a tilt of the head as if picturing something. Or we may have no apparent response at all.

If there is no obvious response, this does not mean the story has failed. Stories bypass our psychological defences and speak directly to the unconscious mind, so please know that on some level the person will have gained some benefit from the time you have given them and the sensory experience you have offered. They have just been unable on this day to express that benefit.

So, let's take an example of one of the sensory stories in Section 3 and work through it.

IN THE ROSE GARDEN

Ideas for sensory resources

- Roses (with thorns removed) to touch, and to display in a vase.
- A realistic butterfly.
- Rose-scented room spritz.
- Rose perfume or body spray.
- Rose-scented hand cream or massage oil.
- A bowl containing cold water for people to put their hands in.
- Rose water and cotton wool to cleanse and refresh the face.
- Hair-brushing and a rose hair accessory.
- Rose-flavoured tea, Turkish delight, rose-scented cocktail (or mocktail).
- Nature-based relaxing music, including bird song and running water if possible.

Read through once without the accompanying sensory prompts.

'In the Rose Garden'
Roses in bloom, it must be June.
A delicate, floral scent sweetens the summer air.
I open the garden gate, which creaks on old, worn hinges.
The rose garden is peaceful but not silent. Bird song and the buzz of bees provide Nature's melody.
Somewhere in the distance, gentle music is playing and it relaxes me.
As I walk along the path, I pause to touch the soft, velvet blooms.
A butterfly dances in the air and then comes to rest on a rose, before flitting off again, over the garden wall.
I find the garden seat and sit, taking a deep, relaxing breath, and dipping my hand into the little stream of water flowing from the fountain.
I feel relaxed and safe, surrounded by all types of roses – tea roses, floribundas, a pale-pink damascene.
I rest here, opening up a secret little parcel of tissue paper to reveal a sweet treat, all for me.
I always find a little piece of heaven, here in the rose garden. *Why don't you join me?*

Long pause… Watch for any responses to the story.
Now read through a second time with the accompanying sensory prompts.

'Let's have that again…'
Roses in bloom, it must be June. *[Say brightly, then pause, make eye contact.]*

A delicate, floral scent sweetens the summer air. *[Spray the room spritz around the room.]*

I open the garden gate, which creaks on old, worn hinges. *[Make the sound effect.]*

The rose garden is peaceful but *not* silent. Bird song and the buzz of bees provide Nature's melody. *[Start playing the music, which includes bird song.]*

Somewhere in the distance, gentle music is playing and it relaxes me. *[Pause and make the gesture of listening, cupping your ear.]*

As I walk along the path *[pat a table or your leg to make the sound of footsteps]*, I pause to touch the soft, velvet blooms… *[Give the person a rose to hold and encourage them to touch and explore it.]*

A butterfly dances in the air and then comes to rest on a rose, before flitting off again, over the garden wall. *[Hold the butterfly and mime it flying before coming to land on the rose the person is holding and then moving off again.]*

I find the garden seat and sit, taking a deep, relaxing breath, and dipping my hand into the little stream of water flowing from the fountain. *[Introduce the bowl of water and encourage the person to move their fingers in the water, before carefully drying their hands on a towel.]*

I feel relaxed and safe, surrounded by all types of roses – tea roses, floribundas, a pale-pink damascene. *[Offer the person a hand massage with rose-scented oil. Ensure all oil is removed with a towel so that their hands aren't slippery after the massage.]*

I rest here, opening up a secret little parcel of tissue paper to reveal a sweet treat, all for me. *[Time for the Turkish delight and whatever drink you have chosen to offer.]*

I always find a little piece of heaven, here in the rose garden.

As you can see, the second reading with the activities added in will take considerably longer and will feel to us like it is taking a long time. We will be feeling the pull to get to the end of the story. We don't like the unfinished. But we will get there, just much, much more slowly.

If the person we are reading to falls asleep, as they might do when having the hand massage, then we should complete the story anyway, just as we would have when they were awake. Their unconscious mind will still hear and absorb it. And no one likes an unfinished story!

Some of the stories work better being read through once, with all of the sensory stimuli added in as you go; others lend themselves more to being read through once at the beginning of the Namaste Care session to create the mood and theme for the session, and then read a second time with the accompanying sensory stimuli. You could also use the stories just at the beginning of a session with one read-through to introduce the theme of the session. This would allow for a less structured exploration of the sensory experiences being offered. It is very much up to the person planning the session to decide how best to deliver the story, depending on the needs of the person/group living with dementia.

As Clarissa Pinkola Estés (1992, p.20) reminds us: 'Stories set the inner life in motion, and this is particularly important where the inner life is frightened, wedged and cornered.'

Each person we approach to share Namaste Care with has lived a rich life. What better way to honour that life than to give them our time? Just about the greatest honour I can think of is sharing precious moments with someone as they approach the end of their life. It can be an emotional journey for us as carers to be in that space with someone, and so my hope for the sensory stories is to provide us with a firm anchor to centre ourselves as we do this work, and to provide a spark of joy for each person on their dementia journey.

REFERENCES

Estés, C.P. (1992) *Women Who Run with the Wolves: Myths and Stories of the Wild Woman Archetype.* New York, NY: Ballantine Books.

Griffin, J. and Tyrrell, I. (2003) *Human Givens: A New Approach to Emotional Health and Clear Thinking.* Chalvington: Human Givens Publishing.

Leighton, R., Oddy, C. and Grace, J. (2016) 'Using sensory stories with individuals with dementia.' *Australian Journal of Dementia Care* 5(6), 17–19.

Matthews, J. and Matthews, C. (2009) *Storyworld: The Storytelling Box.* London: Templar.

4

CULTURAL DIVERSITY AND THE NAMASTE CARE APPROACH

Colette O'Driscoll, St Joseph's Hospice and Lourdes Colclough,
St Joseph's Hospice and Macmillan Cancer Support

The UK has a diverse and changing population. Of people in the UK living with dementia, 33 per cent are from Black and Asian Minority Ethnic (BAME) communities; that is, around 25,000 people in the UK – a number expected to double by 2026. Alzheimer's Research suggests BAME communities face both a delay in dementia diagnosis and also barriers to accessing services (Fortescue 2019).

East London is one of the most culturally, ethnically and religiously diverse areas in the UK, and Namaste Care in East London has addressed some of the above issues by providing BAME communities with information about dementia and signposting to other support services that may be available to them.

It is both timely and a privilege to be given the opportunity to share our unique experience of delivering Namaste Care in East London. We do this in part through a number of case studies which illustrate the impact both on the person living with dementia and on the carer/family member(s), as well as the impression left on the volunteer. The outcomes of Namaste Care on all three – the person living with dementia, the carer and the volunteer – are equally meaningful and significant.

After seeing her uncle with dementia pass away in a nursing home, S was determined she was going to look after her father, Mr B, at home, and she cared for him alone 24/7 with little or no support.

Mr B had arrived from Jamaica aged 16 years with his older brother.

He loved music, from reggae to opera, and took great pride in his clothes. He was a tailor by profession and looking smart was important to him.

When the volunteer first visited Mr B, he was house-bound, isolated and non-communicative. The volunteer came with a playlist of music that he liked, and through her own enthusiasm she encouraged him to enjoy the music by chair dancing and foot tapping. They would also look at photos of him as a young man and he would smile and try to communicate.

S remarked: 'Namaste Care opened up my world, but also my dad's world. We welcomed this jovial volunteer into our home, and we both looked forward to her visits.'

The impact on the volunteer was equally meaningful. She described in detail the changes she had witnessed in Mr B and his daughter from the beginning of the sessions to the end and talked about how honoured she felt to be part of this transition.

RELAXED, RECEPTIVE, RESOURCEFUL

Namaste Care is underpinned by person-centred care provided by resourceful and creative volunteers who are willing to experiment and try out new activities. Many ideas discussed did not work but just as many were incredibly valuable.

Volunteers discussed how some Namaste Care sessions could be difficult, with little response from the person with dementia and tense and anxious family members hovering around, which left the volunteer feeling inadequate. However, by working together in share and reflect sessions, solutions and creative ideas were explored for activities, confidence was built and the volunteers went away with the intention to make a meaningful connection. A volunteer commented:

> It's hard to end sessions sometimes, a real wrench because of the emotional connection – if working well. If not, it can be a relief to end!

For Namaste Care to be delivered in a person-centred way, the volunteer/carer needs to possess the following personal qualities, particularly when working with individuals from BAME communities:

- a relaxed approach
- openness
- receptiveness
- creativity

- resourcefulness
- resilience
- ability to leave assumptions behind
- good listening skills
- good communications skills.

At Namaste Care East London we have volunteers who possess these qualities in abundance and they have provided the inspiration and subsequent success stories which have led to our projects being expanded across East London – from the more affluent City of London to the deprived London Borough of Newham. Our volunteers have been able to support people living with dementia from across these diverse boroughs, meeting their individual needs through a personalized approach to Namaste Care.

PREPARATION

It can be daunting to enter the home of a family with a different culture, background, religion and/or language to one's own, and where the person being visited is at the end of life. If the volunteer displays any anxiety or worries, this can quickly be picked up by the person with dementia and/ or their family. Volunteers are therefore encouraged to take time to relax and prepare themselves before the session. This can be difficult in our busy world as many volunteers are juggling work, studying or family commitments. However, sometimes all they can or need to do is to take a couple of minutes before they knock on the door to pause and breathe mindfully, to let go of whatever worries are on their mind, and to try to be in the moment. One volunteer described this beautifully:

> Part of relaxation is allowing yourself to meet the
> person as they are, to see and be seen.

It is important to acknowledge that we all make judgements and assumptions about other people, cultures and ethnicities. The Namaste Care training encourages volunteers to leave any prejudices and assumptions they may have at the door when entering someone's home for the first time. A volunteer put it this way:

> As I go up to the door, I say, 'My assumptions are mine –
> hold them lightly, soften and see what emerges.'

Volunteers have the opportunity to explore these assumptions/prejudices at the monthly Share and Reflect meetings for volunteers. Creating a safe space in the monthly meetings can allow the group to unpick any issues arising in the Namaste session. This should be a safe place to explore fears, judgements and any issues which may be barriers to working well with the person with dementia or their family. Listening and communication are key parts of the Namaste Care training programme. In order to listen effectively, volunteers are trained to suspend judgements and 'be with' the person with dementia and their carer.

LIFE STORIES

Gathering a comprehensive background history on the person living with dementia from family, friends, carers and health professionals is key in a Namaste assessment. Kitwood (1997) and Brooker (2007) stressed the importance of the unique identity, biography and individual needs to provide quality care that is person-centred.

> HL was an African man with end-of-life care needs. He was matched with a Namaste volunteer who was able to play his choice of religious music in his mother tongue (via YouTube) while she massaged his feet. In discussion with nursing staff we gleaned information about his cultural background – the tribe he came from, and the drum beat of his specific tribe (the wonders of Google!). This provided the soothing sounds which encouraged him to open his eyes and allow a slow smile of contentment and joy to spread across his face.

It can be crucial to help build life stories and understand the sometimes complicated backgrounds of immigration. Some people will have crossed various continents, speak multiple languages and may have lived a more varied life abroad than is known to the family. One carer regretted not finding out more about her father sooner:

> *I wish I'd asked my dad more about what he did in India – his degree, his jobs and his life there. I don't even know what he studied and now it's too late, and I will never know.*

Truswell and Tobert (2020) state that dementia can return individuals to earlier ideas of self, identity and nationality; often people return to speaking their mother tongue. All these facets of their experience make it challenging for the volunteer to gather background history and connect with the person with dementia. However, as our case studies illustrate, experiences of using the Namaste Care approach were enhanced when some prior research was conducted: doors were unlocked, memories found, drums started beating and feet started tapping.

MEANINGFUL ACTIVITIES

When thinking about activities and encouraging meaningful engagement, a person's religion, nationality or culture are likely to have a major influence on their preferred music, food, clothes and everyday routines (Moriarty, Sharif and Robinson 2011). The volunteer's willingness to be creative and resourceful is vital. However, questions can be challenging for people with dementia. Moriarty and colleagues suggest that showing pictures of a country, symbols of a religion or possibly objects related to that culture might prompt different responses. A rice bowl, Chinese fabrics or a picture of a rickshaw might provoke memories for a person from China or Hong Kong. Spices, saris or Bollywood star pictures could be good starting points for someone from India. Volunteers working with Namaste Care use all these strategies, and very successfully. Most of them were *not* from the same culture or background as the person living with dementia they were matched with; however, their willingness to learn and put in the time to do research reaped huge rewards.

> MR was an Indian man from the Gujarat. He had advanced dementia and had lost most of his language abilities. He was matched with a volunteer from a different cultural background who shared his interest in cycling. The volunteer provided hand massage, which MR seemed to enjoy, and he researched and played qawwali music, which MR loved, and this created a wonderful bond between them. The volunteer also provided a listening ear to his wife who was feeling stressed. He encouraged her to return to yoga, which she did and found it helped her to relax.

Of course, if you have a volunteer who speaks the same language and is from the same culture as the person with dementia, it can really work well. One volunteer delivered several sessions before the person with dementia she was matched with passed away:

> *I spoke Bengali. I felt like I was one of the family and*
> *I was privileged to be invited to the funeral.*

On the other hand, some families have specifically asked not to be matched with someone from their own community. In some cases, this may be because of feeling ashamed that there is dementia in the family and not wanting their community to know.

Health professionals sometimes feel uncomfortable working with people whose religions they are not knowledgeable about. Sometimes they wait before they can match someone with a similar background, but our experience shows volunteers from differing cultures and backgrounds who do their research can have as huge an impact as anyone else.

SUPPORTING THE FAMILY CARERS

According to Alzheimer's Research UK, one-third of people from BAME communities believe dementia is a normal part of ageing (Fortescue 2019). The Namaste service can play an important part in informing carers as to what dementia is and providing ideas for how to support their family member. When Namaste Care was rolled out in East London in people's own homes, the crucial and often invisible role of carers became apparent, as did the impact Namaste Care would have on them.

Truswell and Tobert (2020) found that faith organizations rarely provide any support when individuals from BAME communities with a diagnosis of dementia are isolated from the extended family and their community. Namaste Care has been able to fill this void with emotional and practical support for the carer as well as the person living with dementia.

> AB was a Caribbean woman in her 90s who was living with dementia and had end of life care needs. Her Namaste volunteer would bring lavender wax and a diffuser to the session to create a calm and caring environment. She would then massage AB's legs and arms and chat to her as she worked her magic, whilst playing her favourite music.
>
> AB's daughter said the carers could tell when she had had a Namaste session, as she was more relaxed and less rigid, and therefore easier to move and turn. She described her mother, as being 'blissed out' during the Namaste sessions.

Entering someone's home is like entering their world; it is a privilege and a responsibility. Namaste is an approach which involves working through often complicated family dynamics, as well as ensuring that the carer/family are as supported as the person with dementia. Supporting a person living with dementia who has been traumatized at an early age means that as their dementia progresses, they can return to that traumatic time in their life and re-live it. This can be upsetting not only for the person re-living the trauma but for their loved ones and family members.

> MN was a *Kindertransport* child who arrived in London as a ten-year-old. Now in her 90s, with late-onset dementia, she was re-living the trauma and feeling of being abandoned from when she was wrenched from her parents, who promised they would all be reunited again. The Namaste volunteer had an understanding and sensitivity around Jewish children's experiences from the Holocaust. She held her hand, contained her distress, provided comfort and listened to her repeat her story.

This may have some parallels with a small cohort of older people in East London who survived two World Wars, were evacuated and lost parents. Their experiences are not identical but have some similarities. Evans (2004) highlights the need to understand the person's own perspective of the event rather than drawing conclusions based on the assumption of early separation. This also emphasizes the need for a person-centred approach that cuts across all communities.

Truswell and Tobert (2020) suggest that most BAME families have a lack of awareness of services and are often working with shame, denial and community stigma around the diagnosis of dementia of a member of their family.

Of course, this is not the case for all BAME families. Some volunteers were able to support and connect with carers and family members and make a meaningful difference – often through signposting or simply spending time listening to them and seeing them as individuals. For example, one volunteer regularly took cardboard in for a carer who made toy figurines; he showed the volunteer his work and they chatted regularly.

The Namaste Care service for people living at home aims to encourage carers to introduce Namaste activities into a daily routine with the person living with dementia. In reality, however, this does not often happen. Families are frequently busy 'doing' when the volunteer enters the house and are just grateful for a break during the Namaste session, often using the time to catch up on other jobs. However, the volunteers can also support the family by spending some time with the carer – talking about dementia, helping to dispel any myths or misunderstandings, providing information or signposting to other services; thus, carers have an opportunity to offload their worries, have a cry or speak the unspeakable. One carer spoke to the volunteer about the shame she felt, and how she wanted to keep the fact that her mum had dementia within the family and not let anyone else know.

When one volunteer tried to engage with her 'match', the carer said, 'There's no point in doing that; they can't do that.' Nevertheless, the volunteer persisted. She succeeded in developing trust and building a relationship with that person, enabling them to do things and encouraging them to express themselves. At the end of one Namaste session the volunteer reported, 'It's joyful to see that – those moments where a carer might say "There's my mum." The family gets to see those subtle changes – and that gives me joy.'

CONCLUSION

Working with Namaste Care and BAME communities in East London has been a wonderful opportunity to experience so many traditions, cultures, memories and moving stories from around the world. Working with BAME communities is like working with any community. However, it is important to do your research – it will pay huge dividends. It is necessary to give yourself permission to be creative, take risks, make mistakes and be curious. The Namaste Care in the community model was first rolled out in East London, where doors opened. Forgotten histories were found and shared with grandchildren through memory boxes; photos were dug out; and complicated layers of immigration were unfolded – from *Kindertransport* to African chiefs. The matches and stories from the case studies illustrate the power of the Namaste approach: leaving personal judgements at the door, being open and curious, and finding a way to make a connection.

Volunteers crossed cultural and religious boundaries because they were willing to suspend their sense of self and enter a new world. In return, they were gifted with a wonderful connection to people living with dementia and their carers, as well as the realization that they brought a positive and unique contribution to that family.

REFERENCES

Brooker, D. (2007) *Person-Centred Dementia Care: Making Services Better.* London: Jessica Kingsley Publishers.

Evans, S. (2004) 'Attachment in Old Age: Bowlby and Others.' In S. Evans and J. Garner (eds) *Talking Over the Years: A Handbook of Dynamic Psychotherapy in Older Adults.* London: Routledge.

Fortescue, A. (2019) 'Dementia: Third of BAME people see condition as inevitable, says charity.' *Sky News.* Available at https://news.sky.com/story/dementia-third-of-bame-people-see-condition-as-inevitable-says-charity-11748373, accessed on 5 January 2021.

Kitwood, T. (1977) *Dementia Reconsidered: The Person Comes First.* Buckingham: Open University Press.

Moriarty, J., Sharif, N. and Robinson, J. (2011) 'Black and minority ethnic people with dementia and their access to support and services.' SCIE Research Briefing 35. Available at www.researchgate.net/publication/233741268_Black_and_minority_ethnic_people_with_dementia_and_their_access_to_support_and_services/link/0fcfd50af852a5a3d3000000/download, accessed on 4 December 2020.

Truswell, D. and Tobert, N. (2020) 'Exploring Spirituality and Dementia.' In D. Truswell (ed.) *Supporting People Living with Dementia in Black, Asian and Minority Ethnic Communities: Key Issues and Strategies for Change.* London: Jessica Kingsley Publishers.

RECOMMENDED READING

Age UK and the Race Equality Foundation: Dementia in Black and Minority Ethnic Communities: Meeting the Challenge

Findings from a one-day learning event (Birmingham, 27 November 2013). Although the number of people with dementia in Black and Minority Ethnic (BME) communities in the UK is increasing, research on this subject is limited.

http://ref.hybiscas.com/wp-content/uploads/Dementia%20conference%20report%20 -%20final%201_0.pdf

Age UK *et al.*: Dementia, Equity and Rights

Highlights the main issues arising for people with dementia and their carers in a variety of population groups. These include: the oldest old; young onset; people with disabilities; BAME people; women; lesbian, gay, bisexual and transgender people (LGBT); different socio-economic populations.

http://raceequalityfoundation.org.uk/wp-content/uploads/2018/07/Dementia-equity-and-rights-report.pdf

All-Party Parliamentary Group on Dementia: Dementia Does Not Discriminate: The Experiences of Black, Asian and Minority Ethnic Communities

This 2013 inquiry report brings together evidence and understanding about the experience of people with dementia from the BAME community.

www.alzheimers.org.uk/sites/default/files/migrate/downloads/appg_2013_bame_report. pdf

BBC: Religions

A brief summary of world religions and beliefs.

www.bbc.co.uk/religion/religions

Botsford, J. and Harrison Dening, K.: *Dementia, Culture and Ethnicity: Issues for All*

With contributions from experienced dementia practitioners and care researchers, this book (published in 2015 by Jessica Kingsley Publishers, London) examines the impact of culture and ethnicity on the experience of dementia and on the provision of support and services, both in general terms and in relation to specific minority ethnic communities. Drawing together evidence-based research and expert practitioners' experiences, the book highlights the ways that dementia care services will need to develop in order to ensure that provision is culturally appropriate for an increasingly diverse older population.

Dawood, M.: Dementia Has No Boundaries

A 2015 paper published in *Diversity and Equality in Health and Care 12*(2), 81–82. One of the defining features of some dementias is the progressive loss of short-term memory and sense of place, whilst long-term memory remains intact. For BAME people there is a strong likelihood of dementia and short-term memory loss with the added complications of language and culture.

Jolley D., Moreland, N., Read, K., Kaur, H., Jutlla, K. and Clark, M.: The 'Twice a Child' Projects: Learning about Dementia and Related Disorders within the Black and Minority Population of an English City and Improving Relevant Services

A 2009 paper published in *Ethnicity and Inequalities in Health and Social Care 2*(4), 4–9.

Jutlla, K.: Ethnicity and Cultural Diversity in Dementia Care: A Review of Research

This 2013 review (published in *Journal of Dementia Care 21*(2), 33–39) identifies research which could offer insights into the challenges and experiences of people living with dementia and their family carers from BAME communities.

National Archives: Moving Here

A website hosted by The National Archives which brings together fascinating archival material related to immigration to England over the past 200 years. The site encourages users to contribute their own stories of migrating to England, and now holds a large collection of stories from a wide range of community groups.

www.nationalarchives.gov.uk/education/resources/moving

Race Against Dementia Alliance: Race against Dementia: A Call to Action

A 2015 paper listing activities, actions and examples of good practice for working with BAME people, families, communities and organizations affected by dementia.

www.dementiaaction.org.uk/assets/0002/3943/Race_Against_Dementia_Website_version.pdf

Race Equality Foundation: Black, Asian and Minority Ethnic Communities and Dementia: Where Are We Now?

This 2013 briefing by David Truswell looks at developments in the UK since the launch of the National Dementia Strategy in 2009. It considers the extent to which the strategy is addressing the information, support and care needs of those in BAME communities and ensuring that they are supported in 'living well' with dementia.

https://raceequalityfoundation.org.uk/wp-content/uploads/2018/03/health-30.pdf

Rauf, A.: Caring for Dementia: Exploring Good Practice on Supporting South Asian Carers

A 2011 paper. Bradford Metropolitan District Council.

Rauf, A. (2011) *Caring for dementia: exploring good practice on supporting South Asian carers through access to culturally competent service provision.* Meri Yaadain Dementia Team: Bradford.

Skills for Care: Dementia and Diversity: A Guide for Leaders and Managers

A 2016 practical resource developed to help leaders and managers to support and develop their teams working with people living with dementia who are from a diverse range of cultures and backgrounds. The resource focuses specifically on supporting staff working with people with dementia who are from a BAME background, people with dementia who are LGBT and people with young-onset dementia.

www.skillsforcare.org.uk/Documents/Topics/Dementia/Dementia-and-diversity-a-guide-for-leaders-and-managers.pdf

Cultural and Religious Needs of People with Dementia

From the Social Care Institute of Excellence Dementia Module: Culture and Religion.

https://www.scie.org.uk/dementia/living-with-dementia/keeping-active/culture-religion.asp

Truswell D. and Tavera, Y.: An Electronic Resource Handbook for CNWL Memory Services: Dementia Information for Black, Asian and Minority Ethnic Communities

A 2016 Central and North West London NHS Foundation Trust information pack developed to help clinicians and support staff working in CNWL Memory Clinics in five West London boroughs to provide relevant information to people from BAME communities who are living with dementia. It contains information on websites and online resources providing general information on dementia; links to audio-visual material in a variety of languages; advice and information on working with interpreters; and information on local demographics and dementia prevalence in the five London boroughs of Brent, Harrow, Hillingdon, Kensington & Chelsea and Westminster.

www.researchgate.net/publication/312039059_An_Electronic_Resource_Handbook_for_CNWL_Memory_Services_Dementia_Information_for_Black_Asian_and_Minority_Ethnic_Communities

5

THE ART OF DYING

Dying isn't easy.

Not for the person doing the dying, or for the people waiting and watching it happen. We don't talk nearly enough about death and dying, especially the process of dying, even though it is our one absolute certainty in life. How do we want to die? Where? Who do we want there? Do we even want anyone there? What do we want the atmosphere to be like? Quiet and peaceful, or full of laughter and song?

I have regular reason to reflect on these questions as we support each of the people that we visit as part of our Namaste Care project at the end of their life. One very special lady (well, they're all special) died in our hospice at the end of 2019, having deteriorated rapidly and with the community team struggling to manage her pain at home. In that moment, in her home, looking into her eyes, all she wanted was for the pain to stop.

Once she was transferred into the hospice and the pain was under control, her level of sedation meant that she was only able to give us fleeting glimpses of what was going on for her. So, we did the best we could.

Her husband brought in her favourite music to play and kept the lighting in the room subdued and gentle. Her Namaste Care volunteer visited every day and gave her a hand massage, talked to her and ensured the room smelled gorgeous using a calming room spray. She was given excellent care by the hospice inpatient team, who kept her clean and comfortable. Her husband stroked her hair, reassured her, kissed her face and from time to time she would respond with a kiss back. It was very touching and a privilege to witness. The volunteer and I were there as much to support the husband as the lady who was dying, and he told us it had very much eased his emotional pain. The hospice staff reflected that when they entered the room, it was full of love. It was, in the end, a good death. We had created a safe cocoon of warmth and affection for her to take her last breath.

This particular lady was in her early 60s and so it was heartbreakingly painful for her husband to let her go, at a time when they should have been enjoying retirement together. How many of us discuss in detail our wishes and preferences for when the end of our life comes? When is a good time? We all need to get better at having these conversations with our own families and with healthcare professionals, especially after a diagnosis of a life-limiting condition like dementia.

How we die is our legacy to those we leave behind, and I would like it to be a positive one, not one filled with trauma, doubt about doing the right thing and guilt.

As I deliver Namaste Care training to family carers, I am very mindful that Namaste Care is an end of life programme; the people I will be teaching may not be at that stage with their loved one yet, but they will be at some point, and I know with absolute certainty that the gentle, simple power of Namaste Care and the love it enables us to express will undoubtedly help.

In March 2020, I was fortunate to hear a presentation by Dr Kirsten Moore, who is a Principal Research Fellow in the Marie Curie Palliative Care Research department, Division of Psychiatry, University College London. She articulated themes that I had been hearing from families, and experiencing myself with my own father's dementia journey, helping me to frame and have ways to discuss the grief that family carers experience while caring for someone with dementia and how we can better support them to prepare for the future. Dr Moore is currently working on the Embed-Care study, which is aiming to empower better end of life care in dementia.

Dr Moore described different types of grief which are written about in academic literature. The term I had heard of in the context of working in a hospice was *anticipatory grief*. This term is more often used in terms of someone with cancer and with mental capacity who can be more actively involved for longer in planning and influencing their own care and their death. The term *chronic sorrow* is often used in situations where there is a perceived loss of a lifetime's potential, such as in the case of a child born with a disability. However, in the case of a carer's experience of dementia, the term *pre-death grief* is used, and can be defined as the:

> …emotional and physical response to the perceived losses in the valued care recipient. Family caregivers experience a variety of emotions (e.g. sorrow, anger, yearning and acceptance) that can wax and wane over the course of [dementia], from diagnosis to end of life… (Lindauer and Harvath 2014, quoted in Moore *et al.* 2020)

Dr Moore discussed the complications in the grieving process which take place in dementia care before death. Family carers will describe the process as a series of gradual losses over many years, so there is no distinct and clear-cut way to recognize the grieving process. There is uncertainty throughout dementia, relating to how the symptoms will progress, at what rate, whether the person can continue to be cared for at home and how long the person will live with the disease (a frequent question put to me by carers). These stressful, mixed-up feelings can include resentment and anger towards the person with dementia, which is often not voiced but can lead to feelings of guilt and self-reproach. In addition, the fact that the social network of a family potentially does not understand these grief feelings or know how to support the family can lead to the carer feeling very isolated and confused. This can be termed *disenfranchised grief* (Doka 2009) where grief is not recognized by others, or where society imposes expectations about what is acceptable in terms of expressing grief.

After the person living with dementia has died, these feelings of grief can be compounded by a bad experience of the person's final weeks and days. Again, guilt can appear, possibly about not recognizing that the person was dying, seeing them in pain and being unable to help them. Add to this the new experience of the physical loss of the person after years of emotional turbulence, and the loss of the carer's purpose and identity as a carer, it is not difficult to see how the carer may struggle to come to terms with not just the death, but with years of stress and worry.

There are numerous issues which can become barriers to getting support and processing grief. Some are emotional, such as denial, avoidance or reality and guilt in asking for help; some are practical, such as having the time to get support. Services may seem to have barriers to progress due to waiting times, the cost of services, lack of continuity between professionals and fragmented services. However, these issues are widely recognized and many charities succeed in plugging the gap in statutory service provision.

There is much about dementia that we can't do anything about and we have to learn to ride the rollercoaster. However, we can prepare as best we can for a good death, and this experience of a good death can have a profoundly settling effect on the family, who are left knowing it was the best it could be.

I will therefore give some suggestions for what we have found from experience could aid a good death:

- Regular GP practice monitoring and review of medications.
- Good advance planning and emergency healthcare plans, which are usually completed with the help of a dementia specialist nurse or practice nurse and which are regularly reviewed to take into account any change in circumstances.
- Use of respite care to enable carers to continue hobbies and social connections so they don't 'lose themselves' in their caring role.

- Finding fulfilment in the role of carer, maybe by connecting with a carer organization or contributing to research.
- Being prepared to seek and accept the support of friends, family and services.
- Promoting the carer's perception of control by keeping them well informed about dementia progression, what to expect, keeping them involved in planning and, most importantly, acknowledging them as the undoubted expert about the person living with dementia.
- Agreeing with the person living with dementia, as soon as possible after diagnosis, where they would ideally like to die. It is not always possible to fulfil this wish, but this simple request will help frame many of the other choices that may need to be made along the dementia journey.
- As the person reaches the advanced stages of dementia, begin using Namaste Care more and more as a way to continue to connect with them and to remember they're still here and they're still in there, waiting for someone to find them.
- Think about what the person would pack in their 'death kit', What would they find comfortable to wear? Are there photographs or objects they'd like to have nearby? What music would they choose to listen to in their final hours? What smells would soothe them? Pack a brush and face cream, beautiful hand creams and room spritz.

The following stories in Section 3 are designed to be read to someone who is close to death, as a way both to help them relax and let go, but also so that the family carer can feel like there is something they can do, as they often describe feeling helpless and like an observer.

'Time to Let Go'

'The Butterfly'

'All That I Am'.

I think in our modern world, we have lost some of the rituals that were associated with death. Rituals help us to know what to do. In many countries, the women of the village who assisted with childbirth were also those who were called upon to tend to the dying. They knew what to do for the dying person, and their presence eased the worries of the family. In many ways, hospices and district nurses now fulfil this role, but it would be wonderful to empower the family to feel able to do some of the tending – to do the rituals, make the closure.

One way to ease the passing of the person may be to explore the use of sacred oils. Felicity Warner established the Soul Midwife School in the UK and trains Soul Midwives or 'death doulas' both in person and online. Her book, *Sacred Oils* (Warner, 2018) was given to me as a gift by a wonderful colleague at St Cuthbert's Hospice and it is filled with lost knowledge of the spiritual use of aromatic oils and, in the context of this chapter, the importance of how these oils can be used as a person approaches death. Warner recommends the following sacred anointing oil mix for the sick and dying:

In a dark glass bottle mix 10ml organic rapeseed oil with:

- *Rose Otto essential oil (3 drops)*
- *Frankincense essential oil (3 drops)*
- *Sandalwood essential oil (3 drops)*

This is a stronger blend than would usually be used in palliative care for massage purposes, but for anointing, a smudge of the oil on your thumb applied to the dying person's chest over the heart area, the brow and the crown of the head, is a spiritual act of release, acknowledgement and devotion. It does not need to be about religion; this is a sacred act of love. Obviously, however, if the person does have a faith, it is very important to involve a priest or imam to carry out the final rituals of that religion as this will help to soothe the person and prepare them and the family for death.

For me, using a Namaste Care approach of surrounding the person with sensory beauty in the final days and hours of their life can only act to ease the emotional pain of all concerned and lead to a good death. It gives us a framework, a ritual. It's the very last thing we can do for this person. I'm not saying it will be easy, but it will be worth it. Go gently and be kind to yourself. You're doing the best you can.

I was again reminded that it is up to us to make our own relationship with loss on reading this beautiful poem, written by Kathleen Linton. Kathleen is Cyril's wife (the subject of Richard Langdon's chapter on music), a 90-year-old force of nature, proactive and devoted to Cyril, who passed away in 2020.

My Ray of Sunshine

I lost my ray of sunshine most suddenly one day,
Although I wished so very hard, I knew you could not stay.
The quiet room, the vacant chair, the empty made-up bed,
The tears, the grief, the anger, all raging through my head.
Until one night I dreamt of you and knew without a doubt,

It's up to me to keep you near, my sunshine can't go out.
When skies are blue and sunshine bright, I'll feel the warming rays
And know the sun is shining still, on dark and dreary days.

I see the rays that sparkle and dance on water bright,
It lightens up my heart at such a lovely sight.
To lie beneath the stately oak and watch the playful beams
As they filter through the dappled leaves to brighten up my dreams.
Just for a time I lost you, my days full of despair.
How could I be so stupid, my sun is always there.

Kathleen Linton
August 2020

REFERENCES

Doka, K.J. (2009) 'Disenfranchised grief.' *Bereavement Care 18*(3), 37–39.

Lindauer, A. and Harvath, T.A. (2014) 'Pre-death grief in the context of dementia caregiving: A concept analysis.' *Journal of Advanced Nursing 70*(10), 2196–2207. DOI:10.1111/jan.12411.

Moore, K.J., Crawley, S., Vickerstaff, V. and Cooper, C. (2020) 'Is preparation for end of life associated with pre-death grief in caregivers of people with dementia?' *International Psychogeriatrics 32*(6), 1–11.

Warner, F. (2018) *Sacred Oils: Working with 20 Precious Oils to Heal Spirit and Soul.* London: Hay House.

SUPPORTING SENSORY APPROACHES

6

SENSES, SCENTS AND SAFETY: ESSENTIAL OILS FOR WELLBEING

Andrea Lambell, Complementary Therapist and
Member of the Federation of Holistic Therapists

THE SENSE OF SMELL

Our experience of life is shaped by our many senses. We are who we are, and we do what we do, as a result of the way we pick up and respond to constant and varied stimuli. For each of our senses, our body's tissues receive countless messages which are sent along nerve pathways to the brain, where they are processed. Here, each signal is sifted for its meaning and, if necessary, decisions are made to act on those meanings. Some signals are processed and acted upon without disturbing our consciousness, while others are flagged up by the brain as laden with meaning. Both kinds of signals shape our decisions, our actions, our memories, and our physical and emotional wellbeing.

Our ability to see and hear are often considered to be the most important senses because we rely on them so much to communicate and to navigate the world. The sense of smell tends to be considered less important by comparison, but it has a fundamental role to play in our lives. It triggers our emotions, provides a landscape for our memories, draws us to our partners and bonds us with our kin. Its sensuous dance, along with the signals from our taste buds and tongue, enhances our lives through the pleasure of food's flavours and textures, and keeps us ingesting essential nourishment. Our sense of smell protects us, alerting us to the dangers of fire, bad food or insanitary conditions.

The air in our here-and-now is seeded with messages to our histories and our souls. Smells spark a connection in our memory – the smell of tar used to mend a road can send through our limbs a little rush of remembrance of that joyful bicycle-fuelled freedom in the school holidays that year when the weather was so hot the road melted; or maybe the smell of freshly baked bread triggers a warmth in the heart which was put there by your gran, who fed you doorstep-sized slices straight from her oven. Such emotions and memories, unique to our own personal experiences, can hit us before we've even identified the triggering scent. It's important to bear in mind the fact that a smell that triggers pleasant reflections in one person can be attached to an unpleasant memory and emotion in another: what if the hot tar smell reminds you of the dog that attacked you on that summer bike ride?

Scent is so strongly linked to memory and emotion because, unlike our other senses, nerve pathways for smell are hard-wired directly into the centres of the brain which control memory and emotion (the amygdala and hippocampus), bypassing the area of the brain (the thalamus) which filters and sorts incoming sensory messages. We sense a smell when specialized nerve endings in the roof of our nose are stimulated by the touch of tiny packages of airborne chemicals. These are volatile molecules: substances which exist in liquid or solid form but are light enough to detach from their neighbours to take flight in air and spark a chain of electrical and chemical reactions along nerve fibres from the nostrils into the brain's core.

ESSENTIAL OILS

Humans have long known about the power of smell. The roots of the multi-billion-dollar perfumery industry stretch unbroken back through time. Archaeologists have found evidence of perfumery materials in ancient civilizations: aromatic substances crushed, powdered, macerated and made into pastes, ointments and incense. From their findings, it's clear that these substances were used in medicine as well as for wellbeing and rituals. Though animal and mineral material also provided a source for aromatic and medicinal products, the plant world was the most abundant, accessible and versatile source. Over millennia, humans have experimented with plant material and harnessed its properties for their own needs, setting the foundations for modern pharmaceuticals. Along the way, methods were developed to extract and distil the volatile molecules from the whole plant, separating them from the bigger, heavier molecules – the fibrous and water-soluble parts, the proteins, vitamins, minerals and other trace chemicals. That extract is known today as an essential oil. Essential oil packs a huge punch of scent because every molecule in that little bottle is a volatile molecule – leave the lid off, and eventually every last drop will evaporate.

Essential oils from an extensive range of plants are widely available and have huge appeal. The word 'essential' might lend itself to the 'must-have' language of advertising, but its misuse in that context masks the real meaning of the word: essential oils are the essence of a plant; chemicals manufactured by the plant's own metabolism for its own particular survival needs. They deter parasites and microbes, attract pollinators and can create a protective barrier in the air around the plant to reduce water loss or to deter other plants from crowding it out.

Plants manufacture and store their essential oils in microscopic pockets, called trichomes. They are usually too small to be seen by the naked eye, but if you look carefully at the rind of a citrus fruit, you might be able to see them. When you peel an orange, the trichomes rupture to release a fine spray of essential oil, instantly filling the air – and your nose – with that unmistakeable refreshing tang. (Don't be surprised if reading this description has made your mouth water – it's just perfectly illustrated the dance between the sense of smell, taste, memory and emotion!)

Different parts of a plant have different functions: roots, stems, leaves, flowers, fruit… So, it makes sense that the different sets of trichomes in each kind of tissue create their own specialized essential oil chemical cocktail. The essential oil of orange peel protects the juicy fruit within from drying out and is very different to the essential oil of orange blossom, which attracts pollinators. This is why it's worth checking the label for this information when buying and using essential oils, to avoid unexpected aromas and unintended results.

Unlike the generous orange peel, some plant material, such as rose or lemon balm, has a very low yield of oil. Their trichomes may be few and far between, or the plant structure might make them very hard to access. There are other reasons why oils are hard to come by. Some plants are rarer than others or grow in places affected by environmental or political factors which prevent sustainable and economically viable production of oils. This explains why oils can be expensive, and why some are more costly than others.

Essential oils are not water-soluble. This property is used in the essential oil distillation process: steam is pushed through a vat of plant material, which cracks open the trichomes within. The oil briefly piggybacks onto the superheated water molecules, and shakes itself off when that steam condenses, resulting in a floating layer of oil on top of the cooled water. (This 'waste' water, sometimes called a hydrosol or hydrolat or 'flower water', has beneficial properties of its own which can be put to use in other ways – it's how rose flower water is made.) Consequently, essential oils only disperse in oily or fatty substances. This is why, when using oils in the bath, it's wise to use them sparingly (six drops is usually enough) and add them to a cup of milk before thoroughly mixing them into the water – the fats and proteins in the milk help the oil to disperse. It may be tempting to think just six drops will be lost in such a large amount of water, but if you shake in a liberal dose of oil before you step in for your soak, the oil will gradually float to the top and form a slick which could irritate your eyes and skin.

Neat essential oils are highly flammable, and deteriorate when exposed to light, heat or oxygen. Find a cool, dark place to store them, and make sure the lids are on tight. The use of essential oil 'burners' is popular: these are ceramic or metal bowls with a space below for a tea light candle. They should be used with caution, however, and avoided if possible. The aim is to vaporize the oil, not burn it. Dropping the oil into a bowl of tap-hot water will successfully diffuse it without the hazard of a naked flame.

Unscrupulous suppliers will manipulate their products to make a profit. Some tricks include stretching a batch of oil by adding man-made chemicals or similar but cheaper essential oils. If your 'rose oil' costs the same as your orange oil, it's probably not real rose oil. There are many stages from the plants in the field to the bottle in your hand. A responsible supplier will know where their oils are coming from and how they were harvested and distilled. They will test their batches using a process called gas chromatography-mass spectrometry (GC-MS). This analyses the mixture of chemicals in the whole oil and prints out a graph. The oil from each species of plant has its own 'fingerprint'. An ordinary consumer doesn't need to know how to read this, but if a potential supplier looks at you blankly when you ask them for a Materials Safety Data Sheet for each oil, or whether an oil has been GC-MS tested, then go elsewhere. The Aromatherapy Trade Council is an independent and self-regulating organization which has established guidelines for safety, labelling and packaging.[1]

Avoid suppliers who advise the routine use of neat (undiluted) oils on the skin, and especially those which advocate their ingestion – they are more interested in their sales figures than their customers' wellbeing. Do-it-yourself advice which encourages consumers to bypass engagement with medical professionals and properly trained and regulated aromatherapists will result in missed diagnoses, adverse reactions and empty pockets.

HOW OILS AND HUMANS INTERACT

Each species of plant has its own chemical composition of essential oils, so each has a unique set of properties. These properties, originally assigned to each plant's oils based on folk wisdom, are constantly being modified and augmented by a growing body of scientific knowledge. Over the last few

---

1   A list of its members can be found at www.a-t-c.org.uk/membership-list

decades, laboratory research in which oils were placed in Petri dishes of bacteria, fungi and viruses has proved their effectiveness in combating such pathogens. It has also established that whole oils can be both more potent than the individual isolated chemical which seems to be the active ingredient in that mixture, while also being gentler on human tissues. More recently, research in real-life situations is exploring the effectiveness of essential oils in managing a range of physical and psychological problems such as pain, sleep, spasm and confusion. Research using technological advances such as brain imaging is also beginning to explain the physiological mechanisms which lead to these effects. The pharmacological and psychological potential of essential oils in the care of people with dementia is an exciting area of research (Holmes and Ballard 2018).

But just because a substance is natural, it does not mean you can let down your guard when it comes to safety. Essential oils are presented in attractive little bottles which draw the attention of curious eyes and hands, so keep them out of sight and out of reach when not in use. They're very concentrated: that tiny bottle can contain the extract of kilos of plant material. That's why essential oils are measured in single drops and diluted in oils, creams or in the air. It's very important to treat essential oils like the powerful chemical substances they are: they can irritate the eyes, skin and mucous membranes. Use them sparingly and mindfully, dilute them appropriately and do a patch test (see panel) before applying them to the skin.

Essential oils are readily absorbed into the body through the skin and those delicate tissues of the mouth and digestive tract, nose and respiratory tract, and the genitalia. The oil's molecules pass through the fluid that bathes our cells and move into the blood stream, circulating throughout the tissues and organs, before being metabolized and excreted through the urine, faeces, sweat and breath.

Some oils are appropriate for controlled use in most situations by most people, while others are not appropriate for use at all – and indiscriminate use of any essential oil is bad for anyone. All substances – both natural and synthetic – have the potential to disrupt the mechanisms that keep our body's tissues, organs and systems in the finely balanced state of stability known as homeostasis. Just like any other substance applied with the intention of a therapeutic effect, essential oils have a 'safety window'. This refers to the range of doses which optimize between efficacy and toxicity, achieving the greatest therapeutic benefit without resulting in unacceptable side-effects or toxicity. A major advantage of essential oils is their large safety window when they are diffused in air: a few drops of essence in a room is an infinitesimal dose of a chemical substance, but the therapeutic effect of memory and emotion can be potent.

The safety window is different for each oil, and for the circumstances in which it is used. For example, the ingestion of five millilitres of eucalyptus oil can kill a child. That is why, in the UK, internal use of essential oils under any circumstances is against practice guidelines. Some oils, such as mustard and cinnamon bark, irritate the skin in very small amounts. Some oils, mostly from citrus fruits, have the potential to harm the skin by intensifying the effects of ultraviolet light. Some can have an effect on hormonal balance. Some oils interact with medications. For example, wintergreen oil contains methyl salicylate, a substance closely related to aspirin, which has anticoagulant properties. Therefore, it should not be used on people who are taking warfarin to thin their blood as the fine balance of their medication could be disrupted by absorption through applying the oil to the skin, or inhaling steam laced with the essence.

That is why the application of essential oils for specific therapeutic intent in anyone with a pre-existing health condition needs to be supervised by someone who has been trained to consider the specific oil or oils, the amount of oil used, the method and area of application, and the person it is being applied to. But, when used and stored appropriately, essential oils can be one of the gentlest, safest ways to soothe and heal. As long as you're using oils from a reputable source that meets safety standards, and the client's needs are central to the choice of oils and the method of application, you have the basis of a safe and effective therapeutic intervention.

WHAT IS AROMATHERAPY?

Aromatherapy is defined by the regulators of its practitioners as the systematic use of essential oils to improve physical and emotional wellbeing. Some people advocate its use as an alternative to mainstream medicine, but trained and regulated aromatherapists must practise in a way that complements and works alongside their client's medical care. The appeal of this natural and sensual approach to wellness has led to the definition of 'aromatherapy' being stretched to extremes. Some manufacturers of a diverse range of products make aromatherapy claims by incorporating aromatic substances into their washing powder, shampoo and floor polish, with no regard to the difference between genuine essential oils or synthetic aroma chemicals, or the element of therapeutic intent. Advertisers who use the word 'aromatherapy' to market bacon may be correct in claiming that the scent of a bacon sandwich can stir memory and emotion, and such a mechanism has been used by many of us to tempt a reluctant appetite, but you'd soon lose that appetite if essential oils had been anywhere near your bacon butty!

An aromatherapist aims to tap into the sense of smell's unique mechanism, and to use it to consciously and systematically engage the client's mind/body self-healing mechanism by promoting beneficial emotions and memories. At the same time, the aromatherapist chooses and uses specific oils not only for their scent, but also for the way each oil works on the body's tissues, organs and systems.

The mind has an effect on the body in a very physical sense. Fear and stress trigger the release of cortisol and adrenaline, which can, over time, adversely affect the normal functioning of our tissues and organs. The damaging effects of an unbalanced, long-term over-production of these hormones can be slowed by reducing their release and promoting other 'feel-good' hormones such as dopamine, oxytocin, serotonin and endorphins. When a client engages with a therapeutic intervention, they are likely to have hopes and expectations about the outcome. A physical response can result when the experience of the therapeutic interaction combines with those hopes and expectations, memories and emotions: feeling heard, nurtured and cared for can be a medicine in itself; conversely, being ignored and dismissed can take the edge off an otherwise useful intervention. At the core of aromatherapy should be the act of caring itself – but the aromatherapist enhances that link between the mind and the body by systematically working with the client's smell-memory-emotion mechanism.

The scents of the oils are coupled to an experience which has positive significance. This coupling is reinforced by repetition, so a specific scent becomes associated with a specific memory which has an emotion imprinted within it. For example, the blend used in a regular massage, when inhaled away from the treatment room, can evoke the same sensations that were felt during those treatments. If done well, those sensations will be a feeling of safety, relaxation and soothing kindness, mingled with the other previously existing positive connotations from the scents which contributed to the original decision to use them.

Like all substances, essential oils have the potential to cause irritation or sensitization when applied to the body. If used responsibly, the chances of this are very small. That's why it is sensible to tap into a qualified and regulated aromatherapist's knowledge of the oils, their chemistry and how they might affect you. The risk of harm is reduced even more by testing the oils on a small area before they are used on larger areas of the body – a patch test (see Box 6.1). A positive test for irritation will show as itchiness, redness or a rash in the area. Once the irritant is removed, the condition resolves itself. In rare cases, substances – including essential oils – can cause sensitization. This is an inflammatory immune response that only happens after repeated exposure to a trigger product. Sensitization begins with an initial irritation that goes away, but the immune system then reacts on subsequent exposure to the same product. This can produce a red, itchy rash that's not limited to the exposure site. A very rare and extreme form of sensitization results in anaphylactic shock, which is a life-threatening emergency.

Box 6.1 Patch test

Mix three drops of essential oil into a teaspoon of carrier oil (such as sunflower oil or grapeseed oil). Dab this blend onto the upper forearm, on an area about the size of a 50p piece. Avoid washing the area for 24 hours. If a reaction occurs, soak a cloth in milk or carrier oil and dab the area – this will help to remove the traces of essential oil and soothe the skin. No reaction after 24 hours indicates that the oil is safe to use on the skin at that dilution.

This all may sound scary, but in fact, the information can be reassuring – it promotes sensible vigilance and the proper assessment of an individual's health history before using essential oils. And that ensures safe practice. Aromatherapists are required to have first aid awareness and, as a matter of routine, ensure that clients who have been prescribed 'rescue' medications have their medicine to hand when they are having a treatment. 'Rescue' medications are prescribed for people who have a history of symptoms with a sudden onset – people with a history of anaphylactic shock usually carry a fast-acting injectable medication, often called an Epipen. Other examples of rescue medications include a GTN spray for people with angina, and a Ventolin inhaler for people with asthma.

The aromatherapist usually applies oils through massage, but they can – if appropriate – also dispense custom-blended products which the client can use themselves to reinforce the scent trigger, as well as employing the pharmacological effects of the oils. Blends can be vaporized as a room scent. The client can also be encouraged to engage in tactile ways with the oils, which has the added bonus of encouraging the acknowledgement of their own body's value: creams and lotions stroked on areas of concern, oil blends dabbed onto pulse points in moments of stress or bath milks to enhance the enveloping embrace of a warm soak. Taking control in this way can help in reducing the physical and emotional effects of loneliness, isolation and touch deprivation.

Written instructions should be supplied with dispensed aromatherapy products. If a person is unsure or unable to self-apply dispensed blends, a carer might be willing to assist, but the carer should be identified and consulted before the product is dispensed, making sure they are willing to engage in the activity and that they understand how to use and store the product safely.

COMMUNICATION AND COLLABORATION

Aromatherapy, just like any other therapy, should start with listening and talking. Engaging therapeutically with the senses of smell and touch has the best chance of success when the aromatherapist knows the requirements and preferences of the client, and the client understands and approves of the planned approach. The therapist does this by identifying the client's needs and expectations, explaining the benefits and limitations of the process, and considering the client's wider healthcare regime. Then, appropriate essential oils and methods of application are identified by combining the aromatherapist's knowledge, the client's preferences, and the care plans and strategies already in place.

When working with people who have reduced cognition and decision-making abilities, the aromatherapist needs to include the people who have the client's best interests at heart to gather this information, and to observe closely for the client's own ways of communicating. Consent for treatment must be established from the client's representatives who have the authority to give consent on their behalf before starting the process, but even with this in place, the treatment must stop if a client indicates in any way that the intervention is making them uncomfortable.

With the permission of the client or their representative, the listening and talking extends to communication with the client's formal and informal carers. In this way, the aromatherapist can be better informed about the existing strategies and techniques being used to meet the client's needs and preferences, and thus design an intervention which complements the existing care framework. Communicating in an ongoing way with the other significant people in the client's life means they can stay fully informed about the aromatherapy intervention, its aims and its methods – and, if appropriate, be given support to engage meaningfully in its delivery. In return, the aromatherapist can get feedback on the effects of their intervention and continually adapt it to the changing needs of the client.

If a client is receiving medical care, the proposed treatment plan will need to be described to the GP to ensure that they have no objections before proceeding. This can be done by letter, countersigned by the client or their representative to indicate that the therapist has their permission to approach the GP to discuss the client. The letter should contain a description of the intended treatment plan and a rationale for the approach; it should also indicate awareness of cautions and contraindications, the measures taken to minimize risk and maximize efficacy, the therapist's contact details and a planned start date which gives the GP time to intervene should they have any questions, objections or suggestions. Then, if no objections are forthcoming, the treatments can begin on or after the start date indicated in the letter. If the client has health problems which have not been discussed with their GP, the aromatherapist will refer the client to their conventional health professionals and wait until these have been explored before deciding how to proceed.

LIVING WITH DEMENTIA

A good aromatherapist follows these steps to give caring, enjoyable treatments which are tailored to their client's needs and aimed towards integration into the bigger picture of the client's healthcare networks and services. An even better one also empowers their clients to take control. The therapeutic use of oils can be a day-to-day pleasure and, with thought and support, people with dementia and their families can enjoy them in a safe and satisfying way.

Self-care with aromatherapy products can be very empowering, and the benefits of tactile input from self-application of creams and lotions has already been mentioned. Their use needs to be monitored to avoid ingestion or inappropriate use. But deteriorating cognition does not mean the end for aromatherapy – there are other ways for people with dementia to enjoy essential oils safely and effectively.

There are many beautifully designed essential oil vaporizers and diffusers available on the market. They can be a relaxing focal point. But they can also raise curiosity and, as a result, pose a hazard, as can the intriguing little bottles of neat essential oils themselves. Keep bottles out of sight and securely stored at all times, and consider unobtrusive ways to disperse the oils by placing the source out of sight before the recipient enters the room – for example, place two or three drops of neat oil in a small bowl of tap-hot water on an out-of-sight shelf, or on a piece of fabric placed on a warm radiator. Let the scents greet the recipient, rather than the objects that contain them.

Room sprays can be a delightful and safe way to introduce an aroma to a room. But when trying out scents for the first time, or when working with someone whose reactions are unpredictable, make sure the source of the scent can be easily removed from the space where the activity is taking place. In that way, you can easily eliminate the essential oils as a cause of agitation if the person shows signs of distress.

Hand massage is one of the simplest and most effective ways to connect with a person, but extra care must be taken to remove any excess product from the hands if that person is prone to sucking their fingers or rubbing their eyes. If these actions are likely, consider applying the blend to a different part of the body, such as the feet.

Medicine measuring cups might be ideal for accurately measuring carrier oils and making blends, but oil can easily be mistaken for medicine. To avoid accidental ingestion of aromatherapy products when giving a massage, blends should be kept in a lidded and labelled bottle, placed out of reach while the treatment takes place, and stored securely when not in use.

Massage wax is a solid product which melts when warmed by the hands. Waxes which have essential oils added to them are commercially available. You can prepare your own wax if you wish to incorporate a particular blend of essential oils. Unscented wax can be purchased and melted, then the oils are added to the wax just before it re-solidifies. It's a fiddly process and needs to be done well in advance of its use. But massage waxes are very portable, and spills and accidental ingestion are eliminated.

The sense of smell is often diminished by the progression of neuro-degenerative conditions such as dementia, and odour identification difficulties are common. But 'smell training' – the systematic exposure to essential oils and other sources of scent – can help you keep the sense of smell you have, and even improve it (Schriever *et al.* 2014; Sorokowska *et al.* 2017). There are even indications that smell training might have a beneficial effect on other cognitive tasks – a study has shown a bigger improvement in verbal fluency amongst people who undertook smell training compared to a control group who did Sudoku puzzles (Wegener *et al.* 2018). The parts of the brain that process the sense of smell are particularly 'neuroplastic' – that is, able to change in response to experience: animals exposed to odours develop an increased number of brain cells, and the connections between them also increase. For a description of smell training, see Box 6.2. AbScent is a charity which supports people whose sense of smell is altered, and its website contains a rich source of ideas and support.[2] Do take a look – you might be even inspired to take part in its Sense of Smell Project – a collaboration between scientists and people with smell loss.

Box 6.2 Smell training

MAKE A SMELL KIT
Equipment

> Four 30ml/1oz amber-coloured glass jars with lids (these can be found on Amazon or eBay, or through essential oil suppliers)
> Some watercolour or blotting paper
> Scissors
> Essential oils
> Adhesive labels.

---

2   https://abscent.org

Directions

1. Cut out four circles of paper that fit into the bottoms of the jars.
2. Put one disc in each jar.
3. In each jar, add a few drops of one essential oil – just enough to saturate the paper disc. Each jar should contain a different oil.
4. Cap the jars and label both the jars and the lids. Be careful not to mix up lids and jars (e.g. putting the 'Lemon' lid on the 'Rose' jar), because the lids take on the odour of the essential oil in the jar.

Tips

- Keep your smell training jars somewhere convenient so that you remember to use them twice daily.
- Keep your essential oils in a cool, safe place – they will stay fresh for longer this way. The fridge would be ideal, but only if you can be sure that the bottles won't be mistaken for foodstuffs.
- Refresh the jars with a few drops of oil every couple of weeks, making sure the right oil goes in the correctly labelled jar.
- Don't smell train straight out of the bottle. The tiny hole in the essential oil bottle won't give you a very powerful smell experience. Also, you risk touching your nose with the dispenser cap, and this might be irritating for your skin.

WHICH OILS TO USE FOR SMELL TRAINING?

The original smell training essential oils used in the development of the kit were rose (*Rosa damascena*), lemon (*Citrus limon*), clove bud (*Eugenia caryophyllus*) and eucalyptus (*Eucalyptus globulus*), chosen to offer a range of aromas.

The oils below are suggested because they are familiar, relatively inexpensive (except for the rose!) and safe to use in this way. You might like to choose one from each category:

- floral: rose (*Rosa damascena*), geranium (*Pelargonium graveolens*), lavender (*Lavandula angustifolia*)
- fruity: lemon (*Citrus limon*), mandarin (*Citrus reticulata*), lime (*Citrus × latifolia*)
- woody: clove bud (*Eugenia caryophyllus*), cedarwood (*Cedrus atlantica*), patchouli (*Pogostemon cablin*)

- green: eucalyptus (*Eucalyptus globulus*), spearmint (*Mentha spicata*), sweet basil (*Ocimum basilicum*).

NB: Ready-made smell kits are also available from the AbScent website.

USING YOUR SMELL KIT

1. Find somewhere quiet to sit. You will need to concentrate on what you are doing.
2. Uncap one jar and hold it close to your nose. Experiment with short sniffs. Concentrate on what you might be smelling. Try not to be distracted. 'Look' for the smell in whatever you are experiencing. Try not to judge. Just be with the smell.
3. You should train with each jar for 20–30 seconds. When you have finished, close the jar. Breathe normally for another 30 seconds, then move on to the next jar.
4. Do this process twice a day for a minimum of four months – think of it as physiotherapy for the nose!

RECORDING YOUR PROGRESS

Once every few weeks, make some notes about your observations scoring from 0 to 5.

Strength: 0 = can't smell at all, 5 = it smells as strong as normal.

Likeness: 0 = the smell is unrecognizable, 5 = it smells 'true'.

Comment: Write down any thoughts that come to mind.

Note: Adapted from Abscent (2019, 2020) with permission.

Caring for the carers is a vital part of caring for a person with dementia. Carers should consider having regular aromatherapy massages and developing their own aromatherapy self-care rituals. There is a growing network of therapists who are working with carer's support organizations to offer subsidized treatments. Ask your local carer's support organization for details. For advice on how to source your own therapist, see Box 6.3.

Box 6.3 Things to think about when choosing a therapist

- Look for a therapist who is a member of a register accredited by the Professional Standards Authority. They will be insured, trained to a recognized standard, follow a code of practice and keep their learning up to date.[3] A recommendation from someone you trust can be a good place to start, but do check to see if they are registered.
- Talk to the therapist first – a phone call can prevent disappointment.
- Consider the practicalities of mobility, access and privacy – do you want to visit them – and if so, will they be available when you are? Do you want them to come to you – and if so, how will you ensure you're not disturbed?
- Let them know you're a carer – they might be aware of services specific to your needs as a carer, or they could have a discount scheme. But before you pay up-front for a course of treatments, try one first to make sure it's worth the investment.
- How long have they been practising – full-time, part-time or once-in-a-blue-moon? In what environments, with what kind of clients?
- What kind of Continuing Professional Development (CPD) have they done since qualifying? What's their passion?
- Let them know in advance about any specific health issues, if you have any. What do they know about those problems? Do they have enough understanding of your needs in order to take steps to prepare and adapt the treatment to you? They should seek permission from your medical team if you're receiving medical care – help them to do so.
- What records will they keep of your treatments? Where will they be stored? Can you have access to them?
- Avoid therapists who provide a one-size-fits-all treatment which requires you to push your boundaries to suit their needs, or those who avoid interacting with conventional health professionals.

---

3   www.professionalstandards.org.uk/check-practitioners

Be open with your network of care professionals about your intentions to use essential oils in your life. Health and social care professionals who work in dementia care are dedicated, knowledgeable and resourceful. Their toolkits contain a wide variety of techniques and knowledge. Awareness of aromatherapy might already be in their toolkit, or they might have reservations about the use of essential oils – sometimes with good reason, as we have seen earlier in this chapter. So much more can be achieved through collaboration, reflecting on the potential benefits and drawbacks to come up with a realistic strategy that suits your developing personal circumstances. Share this book with them, and you're more likely to be on the same page – literally!

INTEGRATING AROMATHERAPY INTO HEALTHCARE SERVICES

Aromatherapy has become commonplace in some health and social care facilities and services, such as hospices, care homes and outreach organizations. But to be safe and effective, it needs to be embedded in the fabric of the facility. There are many different models for delivering aromatherapy in a formal setting: an agency might be engaged by the facility to supply and manage therapists; existing staff might train up and add aromatherapy to their existing duties; a self-employed therapist might be given use of a room, where residents attend as paying customers; a facility might employ aromatherapists on the staff, or manage a team of volunteers. Each model has its own benefits and drawbacks, but some universal rules apply (see Box 6.4). These rules are also a useful guide for anyone with long-term needs employing an aromatherapist as part of their care package, such as those funded by Direct Payments.

The voluntary regulation of aromatherapy is ultimately managed by the Professional Standards Authority for Health and Social Care (PSA) – the same body that oversees the regulators of doctors, nurses and other health professionals. The PSA accredits organizations that register health and social care practitioners who are not regulated by law. Anyone accountable for the delivery of aromatherapy must hold a qualification that is recognized by a body which manages a PSA-accredited register of complementary therapists. The therapist should be on an accredited register, as that confirms that they hold professional practice and public liability insurance, as well as conforming to a Code of Practice and a programme of CPD.

The facility's or service's managers should assess the aromatherapist's role to evaluate which level of Disclosure and Barring Service (DBS) certification is required. They must ensure the appropriate level of DBS check is completed before the therapist begins work, and ensure it is kept up to date at the appropriate renewal intervals.

Health and Safety Executive rules apply to every workplace, and aromatherapy products and practices must not be overlooked when applying those rules. The Control of Substances Hazardous to Health Regulations (COSHH) requires Material Safety Data Sheets to be obtained and filed for each product in stock, including the carrier oils, lotions and creams. Risk assessments on storage and use need to be conducted and documented, and the safety data helps with that process.

The aromatherapy service needs to be included in the wider health and safety culture: colleagues need to keep the aromatherapists up-to-date with health and safety issues which will affect their practice in the facility or service and include them in mandatory training programmes. In return, aromatherapists need to keep their colleagues aware of the risk assessments and practices specific to their role. Special consideration needs to be given to the health and safety of therapists who visit client's individual homes or who work from their own premises on behalf of a health or social care organization. In addition to the COSHH management of products, their vulnerability as lone workers needs to be taken into account, with specific training and protocols put in place to minimize risk.

Information sharing is also at the heart of safe clinical practice. The aromatherapist should be inducted into the workplace's record-keeping systems. They need to be kept fully up-to-date about the client's status in order to ensure that their intervention is safe and appropriate, and the other members of the clinical team need to be kept aware of the aromatherapist's activity. It also allows the team to co-ordinate care. There also needs to be a facility to record the details of each treatment: the oils and carriers used (identified by their botanical names to avoid misinterpretation), the exact quantities of each substance, the method of application, the positioning of the client, the areas of the body treated with the blend and the techniques used to apply the blend. The aims and outcomes also need to be recorded for each treatment.

The aromatherapist should be regarded as part of the clinical team and included in 'handovers' – the meetings at the start and end of a shift which allow the team to plan their work, share information and evaluate outcomes.

If a treatment plan includes dispensing products for the client's use, there needs to be a protocol in place which ensures the care team knows where it is, what it is for, how it should be used and stored, and how to contact the accountable practitioner for advice.

Aromatherapists can spend a lot of time in confined spaces with essential oils, so it's wise to make sure the room is well ventilated and the therapist takes breaks, and drinks plenty of water. This is especially important when they are working with significant quantities of oils, such as batch-blending or decanting.

Box 6.4 Essential oils – the Golden Rules

- Neat essential oils are:
  - highly concentrated
  - toxic if swallowed
  - skin irritants
  - inflammable.
- *Don't ingest essential oils.*
- Keep oils away from children and naked flames.
- Store in a cool, dark place.
- Mop up spills at once and put the cloth in an outside bin.
- Only use pure oils and carriers – source your oils with care.
- Dilute essential oils before applying them to the skin: two or three drops to 5ml of carrier oil or lotion; less for the frail, the elderly and children.
- Avoid exposing the skin to bright sunlight after applying blends which contain citrus oils.
- Don't apply oils at all to the skin of children under two years old.
- Keep naked flames away from essential oils and carrier oils.
- Consult a qualified, regulated aromatherapist before using oils with:
  - people who are having medical treatment
  - people with long-term health conditions
  - people with allergies
  - pregnant women.
- If in doubt, leave them out!

CONCLUSION

Our Cinderella sense, the sense of smell, is emerging from the shadows. By mindfully engaging with it through the systematic and sympathetic use of essential oils, we connect with memory and emotion to bring comfort. By reflecting on what we now know about the sense of smell, essential oils and their therapeutic application, it's becoming clear that aromatherapy has a place in the toolkit of techniques available to us in our efforts to enhance the wellbeing of people affected by dementia.

REFERENCES

AbScent (2019) 'Smell training: A therapeutic technique for people with smell loss.' Available from: https://abscent.org/application/files/7515/7981/5269/How_to_ST_fold_brochure_with_diary.pdf, accessed on 5 December 2020.

AbScent (2020) 'Smell training kits: How to make your own.' Available from: https://abscent.org/application/files/9115/7532/6765/How_to_make_a_smell_training_kit.pdf, accessed on 5 December 2020.

Holmes, C. and Ballard, C. (2018) 'Aromatherapy in dementia.' *Advances in Psychiatric Treatment 10*(4), 296–300.

Schriever, V.A., Lehmann, S., Prange, J. and Hummel, T. (2014) 'Preventing olfactory deterioration: Olfactory training may be of help in older people.' *Journal of the American Geriatric Society 62*(2), 384–386.

Sorokowska, A., Drechsler, E., Karwowski, M. and Hummel, T. (2017) 'Effects of olfactory training: A meta-analysis.' *Rhinology 55*(1), 17–26.

Wegener, B.A., Croy, I., Hahner, A. and Hummel, T. (2018) 'Olfactory training with older people.' *International Journal of Geriatric Psychiatry 33*(1), 212–220.

7

HEALTH AND WELLBEING BENEFITS OF LIGHT ACROSS THE SPECTRUM – THE ENLIGHTEN PROJECT

Paul Chazot and Laura Johnston, Durham University

INTRODUCTION

The Enlighten Project is unique, bringing together multiple disciplines to address the question 'how does the physical environment and access to natural light impact our health, wellbeing and recovery, and what changes can be made to improve this?'. The current focus of the project is the clinical nature of hospital environments, particularly the stark, highly technical, critical care unit. Most of us will, hopefully, never have visited intensive care, but in 2020, COVID-19 catapulted these specialist units into public consciousness, shining a spotlight on their function and design. Stark in nature, often devoid of natural light, these units are constructed of wipe-clean, relatively colourless materials, designed with infection control as paramount. Detached from the outside world, a sense of time eludes us, and more usual variable sensory stimuli are absent. Spending hours, days and weeks in this environment can be detrimental and disorientating to patients, staff and visitors alike. In this alien environment, we suffer a strange combination of sensory deprivation, due to a detachment from the familiar, and also sensory overload, as a result of 24/7 lighting, constant activity of medical staff and alarm/machinery sounds.

The Enlighten Project is driven by the direct personal experience of the projects' co-creators. Dr Paul Chazot is a critical care patient 'survivor' and Associate Professor in the Department of Biosciences at Durham University. Dr Laura Johnston is a public artist/postdoctoral researcher and long-term carer of a critical care patient, with over nine years' experience as a visitor to critical care.

The central focus of Enlighten Project is *light*, and we seek to apply this creatively to improve the sensory experience of harsh clinical environments for patients, visitors and staff. The methods we explore to enrich our sensory experience are applicable in multiple settings and can bring real benefits in the field of dementia care.

THE HEALING POWER OF NATURE

Research has demonstrated the benefits of the natural environment on human health and wellbeing, yet we all spend most of our time in constructed enclosed spaces. Although some spaces are beautifully designed with a real connection to nature, many of the buildings we regularly occupy have limited views out and little exposure to natural light, natural smells, touch and sounds. In hospitals and in the care setting, the experience is widely varying. More generally, in towns and cities our experience can be of vast open plan offices, buildings tightly packed together and of windowless warehouses which, notably, during the COVID-19 pandemic, became the Nightingale hospitals. The result is often poor levels of natural light and a high dependence on artificial lighting to carry out our daily activities. This has a predicable negative impact on our health and wellbeing.

Where the sun does not go, the doctor does.

Old Italian Proverb

It had been known for centuries that light is of fundamental importance to human health and wellbeing. This can be seen in the architectural design of ancient Rome and Greece and, in more recent history, recognized in the practice and writings of Florence Nightingale.

It is the unqualified result of all my experience with the sick, that second only to their need of fresh air is their need of light…and that it is not only light but direct sun-light they want.

From *Notes on Nursing* by Florence Nightingale

Florence Nightingale recognized the vital importance of direct connection to nature and sought to place her patients, as much as possible, in the natural landscape with access to direct sunlight and fresh air. A return to health was seen to be as dependent on the stimulation of the senses experienced in the natural environment as it was on the administering of medical and nursing care. Notably, even the non-visual ultraviolet end of the light spectrum was exploited as an anti-viral strategy in the Spanish flu epidemic to aid recovery 100 years ago, through nurses wheeling patients out of hospital tents 'into the light'.

CIRCADIAN RHYTHM, LIGHTING AND HEALTH

The colour of natural light subtly changes during the course of the day. We have all witnessed the rich warm light of sunrise and of sunset on a clear day and how the beautiful intensity of early morning orange/red hues subside to give the cool clarity of daylight. Beyond the aesthetic beauty of natural light, there are underlying essential biochemical and physiological mechanisms that are produced by this daily light routine, and their vital significance is becoming clearer. The shift to blue-white daylight is a trigger for wakefulness. In the animal kingdom, the circadian rhythm has evolved to synchronize with the sunrise–sunset cycle, playing a large role in sleep–wake function alongside many other important physiological processes that help to keep our bodies and minds healthy and synchronized.

Humans therefore require sufficient lighting during the day and low levels at night and are most sensitive to the short-wave blue element in natural light. The human sleep–wake pattern is diurnal, with the circadian system involved in timings and levels of key hormones and neurotransmitters, such as higher levels of cortisol and histamine during the day supporting wakefulness and alertness, giving way to higher levels of melatonin in the evening, important in sleep regulation.

It is now established that high lighting levels at night, such as that produced by modern lighting systems, both reduce melatonin production at night, leading to poorer sleep regulation and quality, and reduce morning release of histamine, meaning individuals wake poorly energized, with excessively raised cortisol levels, leading to elevated stress and inflammation. Thus, there is now strong hormonal– and neurotransmitter-based evidence that an inappropriate lighting profile during a 24-hour period plays a significant role in how we function and feel. Acute manifestation of circadian misalignment, such as circadian rhythm sleep–wake disorders (CRSWDs), can be caused by inappropriate environmental cues such as light, which in turn affects our physiology. There is growing evidence demonstrating that this misalignment plays a role in disease and many of the largest societal and health challenges, particularly within the vulnerable and fragile community.

This widespread misalignment is a relatively modern phenomenon, causally related to the advent of artificial lighting during the Industrial Revolution. The world we inhabit has altered significantly with far less emphasis placed on sleep and respect for the day–night cycle. What had been known for centuries of the fundamental importance of light to human health and wellbeing has been lost.

In our experience of modern 24/7 society, artificial lighting has become ubiquitous, with television screens and digital devices even finding their way into the bedroom, stimulating us right up to the moment we sleep. In addition to the length of time that we are now exposed to artificial light, the spectral colour of the light has also changed significantly in the past 10–15 years. The optical spectrum of most traditional incandescent bulbs, of the type that Edison pioneered, peaked towards the red wavelength region. Modern, lower energy consumption light sources have now shifted, however, closer to the blue region of the spectrum.

It was reported over 16 years ago that a low-level incandescent bulb would suppress 50 per cent of melatonin production, the primary sleep-inducing hormone, in just 39 minutes. Even very dim (0.1 lux) blue lighting demonstrates a significant effect in suppressing melatonin. This effect may even be higher for the new spectral outputs and their greater associated levels of short-wavelength blue light luminance, clearly indicating a significant inappropriate effect on human physiology through the effect of artificial illumination. With the modern world being characterized by near-24/7 lighting and the growth in the use of screens for both reading and working, the effect of circadian misalignment is clearly an area of growing significance and concern.

PSYCHOBIOLOGICAL EFFECTS OF LIGHT – DELIRIUM AND SUNDOWN SYNDROME

Delirium is a very common, but refractory clinical state, common in intensive care and in the ageing community, with the growing aged population, occurrence rates and hospital mortality rates up to 56 and 33 per cent, respectively. It is characterized by fluctuating disturbances in arousal, attention, cognition, mood, orientation and self-awareness, and arises acutely, either without prior intellectual impairment or superimposed on chronic intellectual impairment. Delirium often initiates a cascade of events that can include functional decline, caregiver burden, increased morbidity and mortality, and elevated healthcare time and costs. Delirium in older hospitalized patients is of particular concern because patients aged 65 years and over currently account for more than 48 per cent of all days of hospital care. The biology underlying delirium strongly correlates with the circadian light wavelength profile, suggesting that disruption of the 'normal' physical environment may be a prime candidate and 'trigger' for delirium in intensive and end of life care, particularly in the elderly.

Sundown syndrome, or 'sundowning', is a common condition experienced by dementia sufferers and is also known as 'nocturnal delirium' due to its similarities in presentation. It is characterized by high levels of confusion, anxiety, agitation and aggressiveness occurring in late afternoon, evening or at night. The exact cause of this distressing syndrome is unknown, but a combination of influences appears to play a part including, impaired cognition, environmental and social factors along with impaired circadian rhythm. In residential care, dementia patients spend lengthy periods indoors with inadequate access to natural light. This has become even more likely in the whole community, with the 'lockdown' scenarios enforced during the recent pandemic. As a result, disruption to circadian cycles is likely. Along with administering antipsychotic drugs, including haloperidol, treatments can include melatonin, sedatives, massage aromatherapy and bright light therapy for dementia sufferers in an attempt to counter the negative impact on circadian functioning.

BRIGHT LIGHT THERAPY

Exposure to 'bright light therapy' is one method used to treat people with a circadian rhythm sleep or seasonal affective disorder (SAD). This has shown modest positive effects to date. The goal for treating patients who have circadian rhythm problems is to combine an internal clock that is set at the right time, together with a healthy sleep pattern. This will allow individuals to enjoy the benefits of good sleep (where memories are consolidated and emotional issues resolved), and thence raise wakefulness, attention, motivation and cognitive performance during the day, together with an improved 'happier' mental health state. Light therapy can help someone 're-set' their circadian clock that is 'stop–starting'. Regular sleep patterns help to keep the clock set at the 'right' time. Artificial bright light therapy can be used to expose your eyes to safe amounts of light for a specific and regular length of time, in the same way that sunlight does. However, bright light therapy, during the daytime, has to be carefully delivered, through considering the human circadian biological clock at different times of the year, and appropriate diurnal light wavelength profile, which is not just about constant bright blue light. The Enlighten programme is focusing on developing an economic system, which delivers the appropriate light intensity and wavelength profile at the right time of the day and night, in an automated fashion, but with a manual override option for acute intervention requirements and individual preference.

PHOTOBIOMODULATION THERAPY (PBM-T)

PBM-T is the use of a low-energy light source to elicit biological effects for health and wellbeing benefits; it covers a wide range of both visual red and non-visual infrared wavelengths (660–1070 nm) of the light spectrum, with many showing consistent positive biological effects on the nervous system. PBM-T has been validated and utilized to begin to tackle a plethora of different medical conditions, particularly in the elderly, in recent years, and the cellular and molecular mechanisms of PBM-T have become understood to an increasing extent over the past few decades. Infrared light of defined wavelengths positively acts on cellular oxidative states in the cell 'batteries', called mitochondria, and stimulates ATP energy production. It has also been shown to regulate the production of an impressive array of biochemical mediators, including key signalling molecules, relevant to the three 'Ns', Neuroprotection, Neuroplasticity ('new nerve connections') and Neurorepair, all key to the ageing process. Reproducible positive effects of PBM-T have been reported in many preclinical studies, and importantly recently in clinical trials, over the past decade, including in Alzheimer's and Parkinson's disease patients.

CREATING A THERAPEUTIC ENVIRONMENT

The Enlighten team works within the constraints of the critical care unit where infection control standards and practical considerations massively restrict the range of materials and objects we can introduce into the environment. Despite these constraints, we are guided by a recognition of three basic needs which, if fulfilled, can enhance experience of such places, adding therapeutic value and improving wellbeing and recovery.

These are:

1. The importance of a diurnal cycle of light and darkness.

2. A view providing a connection to the outside world/nature.

3. Patient control/autonomy – the means to influence/adjust environmental conditions.

Each of these basic provisions is, sadly, generally lacking in critical care units. Such modern hospital units are functional in design, the hospital bed being a platform for the delivery of highly technical medical treatment rather than an intimate space for care and recovery. Patients are passive recipients of treatment and too often there is little consideration of the human experience, aesthetics or the senses.

This was not always the case – medieval healthcare in Western Europe took place in the beautiful settings of monasteries, where patients were surrounded by paintings, sculptures and gardens. Recovery was sought through a combination of natural healing and the nurturing of the soul.

Nowhere more than in critical care do we see the dominance of functionality and clinical priorities in the design of the surroundings. Often without access to windows, patients are surrounded by essential monitoring equipment, with views onto blank ceiling tiles or other patient beds. Light levels remain static and constant, and often excessively bright. Infection control is paramount, drastically limiting the scope for introducing more comforting materials and objects into these stress-inducing environments.

Experience of the COVID-19 pandemic has heightened our awareness of the benefits to wellbeing of time spent in the natural environment and of exposure to daylight. Lockdowns made people more conscious of their surroundings, some observing, for the first time, natural sounds and subtle changes in weather and light that in more normal, busier times have gone unnoticed. Hospital gardens can offer the opportunity for patients to experience this, and spending time in these green spaces can play a powerful role in recovery.

The Enlighten Project is seeking to increase access to such spaces for critical care patients. The layout of these gardens aims to offer beautiful landscapes where critical care patients, lying in their beds and accompanied by necessary equipment, can navigate pathways easily. Surrounded by sensory planting, patients can see the sky, receive direct sunlight and witness changes in the weather. The power of nature can be immense – feeling the sun on our face, experiencing a warm or cool breeze and the scent of flowers can have a dramatic and positive impact on recovery. Patients from a critical care unit can be taken to the gardens for periods of time to assist in orientation and recovery. Such oases of calm can provide much-needed respite from the clinical hospital environment for patients, staff and visitors alike.

Inside the critical care unit, to address the absence of access to natural light and windows, the introduction of electric lighting that changes during day can provide a means of enriching experience. Human-centric circadian lighting systems replicate subtle changes in natural light and are gradually becoming more widely available, beginning to be installed in workplace and healthcare settings.

Lighting levels dynamically change during the day bringing both visual and non-visual benefits. This lighting, developed by companies such as Phillips and PhotonStar LED in the UK, is designed to benefit health and wellbeing, synchronizing our circadian rhythms by altering the levels of non-visual 'melanopic' lux.

High melanopic lux during the day helps to set the circadian rhythm and is shown to support healthy daytime responses such as increased temperature and heart rate, strong appetite, and general improved cognitive function.

PhotonStar

In 2016, a dementia ward at St Mary's Hospital in London was re-fitted with a wireless LED circadian lighting system by PhotonStar.

This day/night pattern helps to synchronize the body clocks (circadian rhythms) of the patients, which is known to reduce dementia symptoms and have many other physical and cognitive benefits.

Circadian lighting is an exciting and rapidly developing area of technology, which is likely to become more widely available in the future, assuming that costs are kept at a reasonable level. Technology of this kind can potentially enhance the therapeutic environment and provide health benefits. This will be the subject of further research and evaluation over time.

When introducing lighting systems of any kind it is important to consider who the space is used by and how lighting will interact with the materials and objects within an environment. Perception of colour, light and shadow varies from individual to individual and, as we age, our visual perception becomes impaired with the result that we perceive lit spaces differently. Personal experience and personality can also influence perception of our environment. Glare can be increasingly problematic for the elderly, and in clinical spaces with an abundance of shiny, wipe-clean surfaces, specular reflection can cause real discomfort. Shadows can be problematic and disturbing in twilight conditions, therefore consideration of overall light effect is especially important. These features may be triggers or 'tipping points' for delirium induction in an already sensitive individual. More even illumination along with matt surfaces can assist in increasing comfort levels.

THE AESTHETICS OF LIGHT: TRANSFORMING THE VIEW FROM A HOSPITAL BED

During a pilot study in 2018–2019, the Enlighten team created a lamp, designed to meet strict standards of infection control, which was installed close to the patients' beds in a critical care unit. A changing ambient light experience was designed to fill the localized area of the bed space which, rather than functional in nature, aimed to enrich the visual environment, creating an aesthetic experience. Patients awoke to warm sunrise colours, slowly changing to blue-white daylight and, in the late afternoon and early evening, the light subtly shifted to warm sunset hues. Despite the many competing factors within this environment, feedback from staff, patients and visitors was immensely positive. Sunrise colours were found to be uplifting and light altering noticeably during the day provided a sense of time.

> ...there were lots of comments from the nurses, coming in every morning on a day shift saying it was lovely to see the orange light and waking up to it was really nice.

> HDU patient

In the evening, a patient commented that the warm sunset colours gave comfort when visiting time ended and family left for the day. The free-standing lamp consisted of a wipe-clean glass globe on a vertical column. The circular globe – reminiscent of the sun – when filled with a subtly changing light had a simple aesthetic appeal that was positively received by patients, staff and visitors.

In addition to the introduction of a lamp, the Enlighten team installed a device that projected a library of images onto the ceiling or wall close to the patients' beds. Using a touch screen, patients were invited to select preferred imagery – both still and moving – thus providing a new view and introducing an element of choice and control to patients. In the absence of access to a window, the projected imagery provided a connection to the outside world, a view onto nature, colour and texture, and a welcome distraction from the clinical environment.

Particularly popular were moving images of natural scenes including colourful tropical fish and the dancing flames of a burning log fire. One patient commented:

> I love to watch the movement of the fish. I have this on constantly – I can watch them for hours!

LIGHT IN THE DARKNESS

In great contrast to the experience of critical care, modern hospice designs recognize the importance of natural light and connection to nature. Walk into many hospices today and we notice the abundance of windows and views onto beautiful gardens. Patient beds can be wheeled outside into accessible spaces often designed to provide rich sensory experiences.

Hospice and lone home residents, however, find night-time particularly difficult, often experiencing hours of sleeplessness and anxiety. Family members also can spend time through the night with their loved ones, and this time can seem very long and very isolating. Transforming the view from a bedroom window at night has been explored by the Enlighten team, with the aim of removing the cold 'black mirror' effect of windows at night. By subtly illuminating the garden, we have extended the view from the hospice bed. Warm up-lighting, revealing the subtle colours and textures of external plants and garden materials, maintains a visual connection (engagement) to nature during the darker hours. Changes in the weather are revealed in the movement of the plants and this connection can be comforting and uplifting for individuals.

CONCLUSION

Daylight and views for patients, care home residents and all of us who spend lengthy periods indoors are vital for health and wellbeing. We must acknowledge that, as humans, we experience our world on a sensory level, and that this experience directly affects our general health and wellbeing. Separation from the dynamics of weather, the changing seasons, the daily cycle of darkness and spectral daylight is detrimental to both the richness of our experience and to our health. Providing access to daylight and the natural world is of course preferred, and providing more opportunities of this kind for patients and care home residents must be a priority.

In addition, for those of us who must spend most of our days inside buildings, the Enlighten Project believe that the creative application of light, colour and visual imagery can enrich our sensory experience and improve our health and wellbeing.

Little as we know about the way in which we are affected by form, by colour, and light, we do know this, that they have an actual physical effect. Variety of form and brilliancy of colour are actual means of recovery.

Florence Nightingale

As Florence Nightingale acknowledged, beyond the visual and aesthetic power of such sensory experiences, there are also real health benefits, with a coherent biological rationale, achieved, through application of circadian lighting, colour, texture and access to nature. Well-designed therapeutic spaces that enrich our senses really do have the power to heal.

8

A TASTE OF THE PAST

Michelle Kindleysides, Beamish Museum

Taste is one our five senses. As with all of our senses it's perhaps something that we take for granted and don't really stop and think about until we start having difficulties with it or lose the sense completely. Food features a lot in our daily lives and most of our social activities. We very often plan our day around eating and drinking; we use it to help us to celebrate, to cheer us up or to commiserate.

A lot of our memories and the emotions attached to these are associated with food and taste; whether consciously or not. Things like family Christmas dinners, birthday parties with strawberry jelly and ice cream, egg sandwiches on the beach, homemade bread on Saturday mornings, our first taste of alcohol and possibly the subsequent taste of vomit? Whether good or bad, our brain cleverly stores all of these away.

When we put something in our mouths and taste something, it's a multi-sensory activity. Without us even realizing it, our brains are taking in information from our five senses: sight, smell, hearing, touch and taste. The activity of tasting something is rarely done in isolation from any other senses; it is an accumulation of several senses all working together. When we taste something, our brain sends signals from our taste buds on the tongue to different parts of our brain through a complex network of messages. A particular area of our brain is responsible for interpreting these messages from our senses. Many other parts of the brain, such as the parts responsible for storing and retrieving memories and those controlling our motor skills, will also be working simultaneously. When we sit down to eat, our brains will be working to interpret lots of information, for example: What is in front of me on the plate? Do I recognize it? Do I like it? Where am I eating this? Are other people around me eating? What does it smell like? Have I smelt this before? Does it smell safe to eat? Has someone told me what it is? What is that crunching sound in my mouth? What is this taste? Have I tasted it before? Do I like this taste? For many of us, our brains do this automatically and incredibly quickly, and usually without us having to think about it.

But suppose there is some damage in the parts of our brain responsible for interpreting our senses that disrupts these networks of messages. Damage caused by dementia, for example. Even if this is only a small amount of damaged cells, it will still have an impact on the speed and efficiency of us being able to interpret and engage with what is around us. As the amount of damage in that part of the brain, and others, increases, these difficulties will also increase. If our brain has difficulty gathering information from a particular sense, it will become more dependent on the information that it can gather from other senses and other parts of the brain, such as our stored memory, to retrieve as much information as possible to help us interpret what is happening around us.

Our ability to taste, as one of our five senses, can be affected by dementia, but through engaging activities that aim to use all the senses, people can still enjoy food and drink and also the social interactions, memories and emotions associated with those foods.

As we age, our taste buds start to lose some of their sensitivity. Our sense of smell can also diminish with age. Our sense of taste and smell have a very strong connection; taste and odour messages are sent to the brain and combine to give us our perception of flavour. The result of our taste buds losing their sensitivity over time is that people can then only taste foods with strong flavours. A similar experience to this is when we have a heavy cold and we're unable to smell and taste certain things. As humans, we only identify five tastes: sweet, salty, sour, savoury and bitter, and we all have opinions on what tastes good to us. For people with dementia, especially as the disease progresses, some of these tastes start to diminish. Bitter and sour tastes stay the strongest, which can very often lead to people craving more sugary foods, so they suddenly start adding sugar to their tea or only want to eat sweet cakes and biscuits. Some people are only able to taste if something is sweet if it's very, very sweet, like jam or sugary sweets.

Another difficulty that people with dementia may have in relation to taste is identifying what a taste is. The food is still going into the mouth and messages are being sent to the brain, but there may be difficulties in the brain in interpreting some of these messages. But even if someone isn't able to identify what exactly the food is, they will still be able to know if they like it or not.

There may be other difficulties associated with taste and eating, such as holding and using cutlery, hypersensitivity in the top of the mouth and, as the disease progresses, swallowing difficulties too. Denture adhesive, poor oral hygiene and medication can also have an impact on people's ability to taste. All of these need careful thought when supporting people to eat and drink and enjoy their food.

Beamish Museum's Health and Wellbeing Team offer a wide range of multi-sensory group activities within our unique 'Orchard Cottage'. This cosy 1940s-style house is full of original furniture, décor and household objects from the mid-twentieth century, complete with an original coal-fired enamel range. Although the surroundings tend to be familiar to a lot of people in the groups, and very often spark lots of memories, we don't make reminiscence, with its reliance upon the recalling and sharing of memories, the sole focus of the sessions. Instead, our skilled team ensure that the sessions are tailored to everyone's abilities and interests and they are able to enjoy being 'in the moment', without the pressure to constantly talk about the past. Much of this therefore involves engaging the senses in every activity that we do.

As with everyone's normal daily lives, food and taste play an important role in the sessions that we run. But we want to ensure that everyone, regardless of the difficulties they might experience due to their dementia or other disabilities, is able to engage with the taste experiences and the associated memories and emotions. With this in mind, every group session begins with that national institution: the cup of tea (or coffee if preferred). As soon as people walk through the door of Orchard Cottage, they are using their senses to help make sense of what is around them. For some people, who may struggle to quickly interpret and make sense of some things that they can see, hear and smell, being able to see clearly a large teapot on a table, covered in a knitted tea-cosy, in front of a roaring coal fire, with mugs, milk jug and a plate of biscuits, can very often put them at ease because it's so recognizable as the activity of sitting down with other people for a cup of tea. It makes sense. This universal way of saying 'welcome' and inviting people to sit down for a drink is a multi-sensory activity in itself. Before anything touches their mouths, people's brains are working hard to pick up on all the 'clues' in the room to help them understand what is happening and how they want to respond. The more clues the better as they all help the brain build up a picture using information from our senses and our stored memories. Adding in the question 'Would you like a cup of tea?', while pointing to the teapot, adds even more information. The person who is facilitating the session plays a crucial role in ensuring that there are plenty of clues available, while also being careful to try not to overload the senses all at once. We could make the tea in the back kitchen and bring the cups through to the table, but then so many clues would be removed. Some people sat around the table are able to retrieve information about what all this means, what it tastes like and also whether or not they like this taste, and then communicate this with others.

For people who may struggle much more with interpreting their surroundings and some of the 'clues' around, it may be the actual taste of tea in their mouths that is the strongest trigger for their brains to retrieve information and then possibly some of the associated memories linked to this. Some people may not be able to communicate verbally if any memories are triggered by this, but very often you can see whether someone is enjoying the taste or not through a smile or through them asking or gesturing for more, or perhaps looking at and smiling towards another person who is sharing a memory triggered by the room and the tea drinking.

The environment that food is eaten in can massively influence how we experience our senses. This is why a lot of thought is put into how people can experience eating and drinking in Orchard Cottage. As a large number of people living with dementia who we work with are older people, we ensure that everything we use is familiar to them, that is, things they are likely to have used in their earlier lives and are used to using, rather than modern equivalents. For example, the teapot mentioned above, the toasting fork to make toast on the fire, the scales with weights on, the hand whisk, biscuits on plates (not in wrappers). As longer-term memories remain intact much longer than short-term memories for people with dementia, it will be the information from these memories, from people's childhoods and early adult lives, that their brains are able to retrieve more easily to help them interpret things in the present moment. We are incredibly fortunate to have the familiar setting of Orchard Cottage, so that these items can be used in more familiar surroundings. Even for people who need to use different cups, or can only drink liquid with thickeners or need to have blended food, the fact that they are in the multi-sensory environment and sitting with other people can often mean that their taste experience is different from their normal one.

The foods that we use and make in the group sessions are also well thought out. We ensure that we use foods that people would be familiar with in their earlier lives. For example: more 'traditional' biscuits; plain white or brown bread, usually cut on the table from a loaf; and sugar from a sugar bowl rather than from small sachets (which are really difficult to open, once you've first identified what they are!). If we are doing a baking activity we make cakes and sweet treats that are really familiar and simple to make, such as scones, crumbles, jam tarts, mince pies and gingerbread men, and we use utensils and equipment from the mid-twentieth century. We mainly tend to use and make sweet things (as previously mentioned, people often need things to be really sweet in order to taste them and for things to taste less bitter). So, to accompany the bread that has been toasted on the fire, we offer butter (from a butter dish) and homemade jam or marmalade. For people who need to reduce their sugar intake, we can offer sugar-free biscuits and jams if necessary. We have some more accessible cutlery and cups too.

Importantly, where possible, we support people to play an active role in the preparation of their food in the cottage. This adds touch and muscle memory to the taste experience. This can range from something as simple as stirring their own milk into the drink to toasting their own bread on the fire, spreading their own butter and making their own batch of scones. Instead of using small china cups and saucers, which admittedly are more fitting for the setting, we use white mugs with large handles so that they are easier to hold and are also much easier to see against the plain blue oilcloth on the table. We use plain plates too, so that they can be seen on the tablecloth and the food on them can be seen more easily. This obviously varies depending on people's individual abilities. Where possible, we are able to make adaptions so that people can still safely play some role in how they experience their food.

As testament to the huge impact that environment and sensory engagement can play in people's experience of food and taste, there have been many instances where people have eaten much more during their time at Orchard Cottage than they usually would at home or in their care setting. People who usually only eat small amounts throughout the day and don't often socialize at meal times are seen to eat two slices of toast, several biscuits and then their lunch afterwards, all while enjoying the company of others around the table. Even within this short space of time, we can help to reduce dehydration and under-nutrition for that person. Very often people will comment on the taste of the tea, saying, 'My, that's a good cup of tea; that's a proper cup of tea.' They often assume that it must be Ringtons Tea, a popular and long-standing North Eastern company. This often leads on to a conversation about favourite foods, local delicacies, shopping – all from the shared experience of the taste of tea.

We're also fortunate at Beamish to have other places where people can experience familiar foods within familiar and evocative surroundings. At the Fish & Chip shop, with its coal-fired ranges, people can smell the chips and the beer-battered fish long before they reach the door. Once inside, they can see the food being cooked, before their hot chips are served in reproduction newspaper with small wooden forks. We've seen people who don't usually eat much devour these chips within minutes. At the sweet shop it is as if an invisible wave of sugar reaches our noses as we walk in. For many people, being able to see all the brightly coloured sweets in the glass jars behind the counter must conjure up childhood memories, a lot of which are associated with the taste of favourite or least-favourite sweets. Again, we can see how lots of different senses are involved here to make that taste even more intense when it reaches the mouth. Sometimes it's the fact of being somewhere more familiar that makes people feel much more at ease and so more inclined to want to eat and to actually enjoy food and its taste. This can then help to reduce the risk of dehydration and under-nutrition.

From the examples above it's clear that another aspect of tasting and enjoying food often comes from it being done with other people. The social interaction around food can be just as strong a memory as the taste of it. As we see so often at Beamish, for people who are feeling slightly nervous and who may be struggling to make sense of their surroundings, being able to sit with another person or perhaps a group of people who are experiencing the same thing might well be the first step in helping them to feel more at ease. Another really important role of the person leading the session, or perhaps the family carer in a smaller setting, is to ensure that they are welcoming, friendly and support conversations between other people. This shared experience of sitting down with a cup of tea can often be a really good place to start. If people feel more relaxed and comfortable, they are more likely to feel like eating and to then also take notice of what they're eating and enjoy the taste and flavours of it. An example from my own family is my grandmother, who now lives in a care home. When she moved in, I passed on a list of the foods that she liked to eat, which they make for her, but she rarely eats much either in the dining room or in her own room. But when I bring her to my house for a meal and make something that I know she likes, she eats every last bit (and I'll admit I'm not the best cook!). This again shows how important the physical and social environment is in helping people to feel more at ease so that they can then begin to engage with their senses and enjoy the food they're eating.

I've used examples from our settings at Beamish Museum to show the importance of taste, how the different senses can combine to produce the experience of taste and how taste can be affected by dementia. The environment that we have is unique, but the theories behind what we do – using different senses, using familiar objects and foods, not overloading the senses, making food and drink a sociable experience – can all be replicated in other settings.

9

CONNECTING THROUGH TOUCH

Susannah Thwaites, Occupational Therapist and Certified PAC™ Trainer and Coach, Tees, Esk and Wear Valley NHS Trust (TEWV)

Emma Biglands, Occupational Therapist and Namaste Lead, Tees, Esk and Wear Valley NHS Trust

With special contributions from Ellen's husband, Tom

As Nicola highlighted in her first book (Kendall 2019), and in earlier chapters here, loving touch is part of the bedrock of Namaste Care and a key ingredient for physical, emotional and spiritual relationships to flourish. However, touch can also be experienced as unwelcome and unpleasant by people living with dementia, so as care partners we need to proceed with caution, using knowledge and skill as we seek to gain and maintain connection with the person.

A TOUCHY SUBJECT

The tactile system is the body's largest sensory system, with the receptors located in the skin and the mouth. As well as developing emotional and social bonding throughout life, it also has a role in protection and safety by prompting withdrawal or avoidance of danger. Due to the different tactile receptors and neural pathways linking with different parts of our brain, theories of sensory integration suggest that light and moving touch is more likely to alert our fight-or-flight response, and slow deep pressure touch is calming to our nervous system (Bundy, Lane and Murray 2002).

As we have evolved, and as we progress through to adulthood, the pre-frontal cortex of our brains has the job of keeping our primitive amygdala in check. Steve Peters' (2012) description of the limbic system being like a chimp that reacts instinctively to things, and the pre-frontal cortex being the human who is responsible for adding in reason and judgement, illustrates this beautifully. An example may be an embarrassing and discomforting medical procedure that our 'chimp' is tempted to not undergo, but our 'human' tells us that the consequences of not going through with it far outweigh the unpleasantness, that it will be over in no time, that the doctor has seen it all before and therefore it is in our interests to consent. Without this commentary and decision-making from our frontal lobe, the fight-or-flight response would be to resist such an experience. This is how it may be for a person living with dementia who has changes in their frontal lobe and whose amygdala is being triggered by some form of touch during care – they react automatically to protect themselves from something they are experiencing as a threat.

POSITIVE APPROACH TO CARE™

All staff at TEWV older persons' mental health services are trained in Teepa Snow's Positive Approach to Care (PAC™) as this gives practical skills to avoid eliciting a fight-or-flight response from a person living with dementia and keeps the relationship as the most important thing. We would like to share some of the key aspects of PAC and how they relate to using touch to connect with and support the person.

Hand under Hand™

In PAC training sessions we put people into pairs and get one person to close their eyes and have their partner touch them without telling them what they are going to do. The room usually fills with shrieks and nervous laughter, but it is also the moment when people start to realize that if we touch a person with dementia without showing them or telling them what we are going to do, it will alert their amygdala as we are often using light touch during care interventions. The next step is to have everyone touch themselves in the same places and see if it makes them jump (which of course it doesn't as when your hand is doing the action it is a closed circuit in the brain and you cannot give yourself a shock). A key principle of PAC is 'doing with' not 'doing to' a person living with dementia and we can do this by using a technique called Hand under Hand (HuH™) to connect with them and use well-rehearsed neural pathways (motor memory) to support them with a range of practical tasks.

In brief HuH can be used for:

- connection and providing reassurance; deep pressure in the base of the thumb releases the feel-good hormone oxytocin
- gaining and maintaining attention; uses the sensory-motor tract of hand–eye connection
- 'doing with', not 'doing to', the person when substituting for loss of fine motor skills when supporting in eating, dressing, brushing teeth, etc.

Visual, verbal, touch cues

Another key principle in PAC is that we always give visual cues, followed by verbal cues, and then add touch cues last to avoid the above scenario of the person being startled. It is important to take a moment to think about how both vision and the ability to benefit from verbal cues may change in dementia.

To illustrate the changes in visual field experienced as people progress through dementia, put your hands up to your face and make a 'scuba' mask with your hands – this helps to mimic the changes to visual field in the earlier stages of dementia, which can also be described as tunnel vision. For the middle stages, make your hands into 'binoculars'. Put them on and notice how you cannot see anything to the sides or what is on the table right in front of you. Finally, close one eye and place your hand as if it were a monocle around the other eye – now notice how you can only see what is directly in front of you, how limited it is and how judging how near and far things are from you is very difficult. We will discuss in a moment how we adapt our approach in PAC to take account of these changes.

When giving verbal cues, we need to be aware that not only the use but also the understanding of everyday language changes with dementia. Another of the exercises we use in PAC training is to get partners to approach one another and say they are going to help the other person to 'dabble their dobs' but give no further information or cues. This aims to get people to realize that we may *think* we have explained what we are going to do and *think* that the person has understood and agreed or consented to being touched by us, and then we are surprised when they have a negative reaction to our 'support'. One change that we can make is to give a visual cue or gesture alongside the words so that 'dabble your dobs' is transformed into 'brushing your teeth'.

Positive Physical Approach™

Teepa Snow (2012) has developed some simple steps, which can be adapted to different situations and needs, called Positive Physical Approach (PPA™). These take account of the changing abilities of the person mentioned above.

When people have reduced visual fields, we need to approach them from the front, from a distance of about six feet, so that they can see us and see our faces. We get their attention with a visual cue (putting our hand up to our face) and then give them some simple verbal information (e.g. we say their name and our name). The next step is to give another visual cue by holding out our hand to offer a handshake. This simple gesture is an automatic social cue that tells the person without any words that we want to come into their intimate space and touch them. If they then reciprocate and offer their hand, we know they have agreed and consented to our approach and can move forward and shake hands. From the handshake we move into a Hand under Hand™ position, which allows us to maintain the connection with the person, and can then shift into the more supportive stance to the side of them to continue the engagement.

The GEMS®: Brain change model

The GEMS model (Snow 2020) focuses on the person's retained abilities, rather than their losses, at different stages of dementia. Snow developed it partly derived from the Allen Cognitive Levels (Allen 1999). By understanding the changes at each level, care partners can match their approach and support; it also encourages us to be in the moment with the person and recognize that GEMS states can change across the day. Our use of Namaste Care has focused upon the Amber, Ruby and Pearl GEMS, which we will discuss when we share Ellen's journey with you later in the chapter.

THE PERSON FIRST...

When it comes to touch, as with all the senses, we all have different preferences, needs and thresholds that have developed in response to, and over the course of, our life experiences. Winnie Dunn's work (2007) on sensory processing suggests that we develop mechanisms to seek or avoid sensation to keep ourselves feeling right. This is why the sensory biography is such a central and important part of Namaste Care. Has the person always shied away from hugging friends and family or were they 'touchy feely'? Did they always need to fiddle with things to help them concentrate? Did they need soft cushions and throws to snuggle up in and stroke? Did they cope with a stressful day by having a hot bath and putting on soft pyjamas? Have they always cut the labels out of clothes as soon as they bought them? As people journey through their dementia, they may be unable to seek or avoid what they need due to changes in cognitive abilities or the environment they find themselves in, and this can lead to distress.

Emma had the privilege of working with Ellen and her devoted husband, Tom, through their journey of dementia together from the middle stages to the end of Ellen's life. Tom has kindly agreed to share some of their story to show how they adapted the use of touch to match with Ellen's skills, abilities and needs at different stages (GEMS®) of her dementia.

Ellen was a feisty lady at times. She was an amazing cook. She loved her clothes, fine fragrance, her garden and, most of all, her family. Working alongside Ellen and Tom was certainly a lesson to me in love and dedication. As a couple they taught me so much about the importance and benefit of unhurried loving touch and how we must listen to the person with dementia and know their sensory biography, their preferences and dislikes in order to get things 'just right'. My involvement with Ellen and Tom was over several years and I witnessed Ellen's sensory journey through her dementia, from when she was able to recognize and respond with words and actions to the time when she needed others to initiate the actions in order to make those treasured moments of connection through touch.

GEMS STATE AMBER

People functioning within Amber level live in the moment; react and are interested in how things look, sound, smell, taste and, importantly, how they feel. People at this level like to keep busy with their hands. Language skills are starting to diminish so it becomes increasingly more important to be mindful to use a visual, then a verbal, then a touch cue to help with understanding (as discussed earlier).

During my occupational therapy sessions with Ellen, I noticed that she was often 'tactile seeking'. I witnessed her reaching out to Tom to touch and hold his knee. She would greet with a handshake or a hug and would touch clothing to explore the texture and comment on how it felt. Touch helped her to make sense and connect with the objects and people in her world. Tom recognized this and he would encourage her to help with folding items such as the bedding, dusting, touching and organizing her ornaments. He noticed a positive effect when she washed and dried the dishes: 'This was very much part of our evening routine. I could see her just relax and become calmer.' Ellen continued to care for her cat, Coco, and would spoil her with her favourite kitty treats. On an evening Ellen and Tom enjoyed sitting together, holding hands.

Our sessions often focused on touch activities. I recall a wonderful session we had sorting through Ellen's many beautiful clothes and putting on her favourite hand cream. She enjoyed taking her clothes from the wardrobe, one by one, organizing them on the bed and touching the fabrics, inviting me to share in her experience. She loved to have pamper sessions with her daughter, Claire. They would enjoy spending unhurried mother-and-daughter time together, washing and blow-drying Ellen's hair and doing her nails (she loved to spend time choosing the colours and having her nails painted).

The aim of occupational therapy at this stage was to encourage and preserve Ellen's fine motor skills. Our support worker made a sensory apron for Ellen, which was a bit of a hit. She would spend time exploring the fluffy pompom and the lace edging and would run her fingers along the length of the silk ribbons. The support worker also offered hand massage, which more often than not resulted in them both being so relaxed that one of them would nod off. These activities all provided the 'just right' tactile input to soothe and regulate Ellen's often 'switched on' nervous system, which helped in some ways to calm her 'fight-or-flight' responses. However, not all of the sessions were a hit... She definitely did not enjoy rummaging through her button box!

GEMS® STATE RUBY

At this GEMS level, fine motor skills are starting to be lost, but strength remains and we start to see major sensory changes. Tactile cues become helpful, such as touching the part of the body to be moved or used, offering comfort touch with care before tasks are attempted, and offering calming deep pressure with a flat hand when supporting with self-care tasks such as washing. HuH™ is a helpful physical cue. It is important to avoid touching too quickly and with light touch as this can be alerting and result in a startled reaction, activating the fight-or-flight response.

The occupational therapy aims for Ellen now were about tapping into her gross motor skills, using big movements. People at this level like to have things to pick up, hold, carry, wipe, rub, grip, squeeze and pinch. Ellen continued to enjoy walking in the garden and would often be outside, gathering up leaves; holding and feeling then in her hands (she just loved it); and, of course, her beloved cat, Coco, still got her daily strokes.

Ellen stopped showing interest in her sensory apron and Tom noticed that she would hold onto things and people more tightly. He noticed that she now needed more support and she did not consistently recognize objects. She was also sleeping more. She started to become distressed in the shower and really disliked having her hair washed. She tolerated being washed with a flannel while sitting, and Tom would support her using slow, unhurried, deep-pressure circular movements, all of the time giving reassuring and comforting words. Move too quickly, Tom realized, and her response would be 'no, get off'. They tried no-water shampoo, which was more tolerable. Both Tom and Claire still shared in the pampering activities Ellen enjoyed: having her hair brushed, her nails done and her favourite creams rubbed into her skin.

It was at this time that Ellen was admitted to hospital and with a heavy heart Tom and her family accepted that Ellen now needed 24-hour care.

GEMS® STATE PEARL

People at this level are approaching the end of their life. Teepa Snow uses the analogy of a pearl within the shell of an oyster. The outer layer can seem quite ugly and hard, and it is difficult to see inside, but when you do, what lies within is something so special and so precious.

It is now important to use both hands to give comfort care and to focus on the relationship, not on the task. Go slowly, keep quiet. When giving touch cues, use firm but gentle palm pressure to make contact and keep contact using the flats of fingers and palms for care. Use circular, rotational movements to help relax the joints and provide gentle care for fragile and dry skin.

Even though it was becoming harder to connect with Ellen, she was still there. Tom recalls a visit to their daughter's house for Sunday lunch: Tom and Ellen sat together at the table; Tom asked Ellen if she was hungry and then shouted through to their daughter, 'Come on, we are Hank Marvin out here' and Ellen chirped in 'I'll hank you,' which resulted in great laughter and joy and is a memory that remains with them.

Ellen enjoyed the visits from the therapy dog and cat to the care home, and visits from Claire for her valued pampering sessions continued. Tom visited Ellen every day. He supported her with eating, sang to her, held her hands, brushed her hair and talked to her. Their connection through touch remained unbroken, despite her being in the advanced stages of her dementia.

My final visit to Ellen was special. She was in her bed, her eyes were closed and Tom had left the room to speak with the staff. I spoke to Ellen with a deep and calming voice, introducing myself first then holding her hand in mine. She responded with a flicker of her eyelids.

I told her she looked beautiful and it was wonderful to see her again. I gently pressed her hand into mine, she opened her eyes for a moment, there was a twinkle, and we connected. It was a fleeting but oh-so-precious moment.

Ellen's journey ended on 31 July 2019. Her final day was and still is, a treasured memory, surrounded by her family, with her grandchildren running around and the chatter of life. Claire remembers holding her mum's hands throughout the visit. Tom and their eldest son, Tom, had stepped out for some fresh air when the staff suggested that they needed to be with Ellen. In her final moments they sat with her, holding her hand, with calming, comforting touch: the final gift of connection and love that they shared with each other.

CONCLUSION

We hope that sharing Ellen's journey has given an insight into how the focus of Namaste Care, and how we use touch to connect, need to be flexible and adapted as the person's needs and abilities change whilst still holding true to the person they are and were before dementia came uninvited into their life.

REFERENCES

Allen, C.K. (1999) *Structures of the Cognitive Performance Modes*. Ormond Beach, FL: Allen Conferences, Inc.

Ayres, A.J. (2005) *Sensory Integration and the Child* (2nd edn). Los Angeles, CA: Western Psychological Services.

Bundy, A.C., Lane, S.J. and Murray, E.A. (2002) *Sensory Integration Theory and Practice* (2nd edn). Philadelphia, PA: F.A. Davis Company.

Dunn, W. (2007) *Living Sensationally: Understanding Your Senses*. London: Jessica Kingsley Publishers.

Kendall, N. (2019) *Namaste Care for People Living with Advanced Dementia: A Practical Guide for Carers and Professionals*. London: Jessica Kingsley Publishers.

Peters, S. (2012) *The Chimp Paradox: The Mind Management Program to Help You Achieve Success, Confidence, and Happiness*. New York, NY: TarcherPerigee.

Snow, T.L. (2012) *Dementia Caregiver Guide: Teepa Snow's Positive Approach Techniques for Caregiving, Alzheimer's and Other Forms of Dementia*. Mason, OH: Cedar Village Retirement Community.

Snow, T. L. (2020) *The GEMS®: Brain Change Model*. Available at https://teepasnow.com/about/about-teepa-snow/the-gems-brain-change-model, accessed on 6 January 2021.

10

THE UNIVERSAL JOY OF MUSIC

Richard Langdon, Namaste Care Volunteer

If music be the food of love, play on.

Shakespeare: *Twelfth Night*

We live with music around us. Music provides a stimulus to our thoughts, inspiration in what we do, memories of happy and sad times, and can fill us with emotion – often emotional memories.

One does not have to have hearing to enjoy it. It can be felt. Dame Evelyn Glennie, the percussionist, has been profoundly deaf since she was 12 years old. She feels the music. She plays in bare feet to sense the music the better. She will tell you she listens with all parts of her body. And so should we.

For those living with advanced dementia, music is often a catalyst to their awakening. Find the right music and watch such a person come alive. Some who have been spending their time in silence, heads bowed, unfurl like a flower with a look of real pleasure on their faces and communication is there in response to music.

It is not just the patient who benefits, but also those close to him or her. It gives them so much pleasure to see their loved one, whom they spend hours caring for, smile, come alive and be happy. It can reawaken that bond between husband and wife – together for many decades but for whom dementia has begun to cut one of them off and cause them to withdraw – when music opens the door again and the love and happiness pour out. Watching this happen is itself an emotional experience, but a happy one.

There are videos online showing Namaste Care at work using music.[1] You watch them with tissues close at hand. But to physically see it happen, be

---

1   For example, 'Music and Dementia: The Power of Music on Alzheimer's'. Available at www. youtube.com/watch?v=6BAFB5TtO_w.

present, to use it to help, is not something to forget. Yet it is a simple pleasure and a simple one to fulfil. It needs to be employed more often.

Yes, music is the food of love. Very much so. How do we introduce it?

I was matched with a patient with advanced dementia named Cyril. He was in his 90s. It has been explained in other chapters that on an initial visit there is a getting-to-know you period. Notes are prepared – 'My Namaste Care' being a sensory life story format we use. As much background detail as possible is obtained, right back to childhood, for therein lies the source of conversation, of reawakening memories. Along the way, a patient, or his or her carer, is asked about what music is liked. Often, initially it is the carer who provides the answers.

Sitting with a patient, holding hands, talking about their past – getting married, having a family, work, where they have lived – is not something to rush; it can be tiring for the patient. Introduce well-liked music and there is renewed life. It is a break from the questions. It is calming, it is exciting.

It is not difficult to introduce. Just find out what the patient likes to listen to and let it develop from there. On my visit to Cyril, I found out he liked Gilbert and Sullivan. On the mention of them he burst into song singing, 'I've got a little list' from *The Mikado*, followed by 'Three little maids from school'. That gave me the idea to develop this further and back home I downloaded *The Mikado* and set up a playlist on my iPhone. I have a subscription to Apple Music, which, for very little cost, opens the door for me to access just about all music. I am sure those who use Spotify or other streaming services can do the same. It is about the cost of a music CD each month.

Back I went on my next visit and took with me a portable speaker. There are many types available, some of which are relatively inexpensive. Such speakers provide a much better quality sound than the iPhone on its own does, and also better control of volume. Remember that often the patient we visit may be hard of hearing, so you may need some volume. Back I went with Gilbert and Sullivan and some other music I thought Cyril would like. His wife, Kathleen, went off to make us a cup of coffee and I put the music on, turned up the volume and watched as Cyril came alive with a look of sheer pleasure, beating time with the music and singing along with it.

I also found out he liked organ music, so on another occasion I played the first part of Bach's *Toccata and Fugue in D Minor*. That's the piece where in the first dozen bars or so the organist hits bottom F on the pedals and makes everything, including your bones, vibrate. Again, the response from Cyril was tremendous. This then developed into other music to enjoy and lift Cyril's spirits, as well as Kathleen's of course. She was delighted to see him so happy. This happiness and change is not a momentary one. It lasts for a good length of time following the visit.

All was good with this until COVID-19 hit the country. I could no longer visit but I could ring regularly. Kathleen always answered the phone and would put him on the line with 'It's Richard for you.' 'I don't know him, do I?' Cyril would say, followed by Kathleen's response, 'You know, Richard, the man that plays you music.'

As I write these pages the lockdown continues and my regular phone calls to Cyril and Kathleen continue, but she tells me they now have music sessions where she finds music and plays it on the radio or some other device and it provides an enjoyable and happy time. It only took the one visit where I brought some music with me to unlock this door, and now it is not possible to lock it again. Kathleen tells me they listen to more and more music (I have been able to expand the range of music in Cyril's special playlist), which is helpful not only for him but to his wife as well. In a sense, it is better than giving him pills. Music will continue to give immense pleasure, relief and support; it will continue to open up Cyril, and any other person with his needs, to a level that possibly was not achievable before. Mankind has always had music and used it for effect and pleasure, yet often it is forgotten as a simple tool for relief.

To do this is simple and cheap.

What do you need?

- A mobile phone or music device such as an iPod or iPad to which you can save music. Most of us now have mobile phones that will do this. Indeed, they do everything bar making the coffee.
- If you have CDs, you could copy them onto the phone. (If you do not know how, there is bound to be someone in your family who does!)
- Even better is a subscription to something like Apple Music or Spotify – with that you just find the music you want and download it straight in. Of course, you will have done your research and found out what your patient likes but it's fine to experiment and add something different.

I have in mind to introduce a piece of music by a French composer called Lefébure Wély. He named it 'Sortie in E Flat'. It is a piece of organ music that is vibrant, cheerful and sounds like something you used to hear coming from the steam engines in a fairground. I am certain Cyril will love it. I can picture him now, strumming with his fingers and involving himself with the sound.

Simple really. Music is the food of love. Better than a paracetamol. Its presence improves everything and in particular the life of your match and their family. Our task is not to cure, but to provide relief and comfort, to enable a better quality of life, to generate happy responses and to make the effects of dementia more palatable; and at the same time, knowing what the end result will be, to smooth that passage for all. Music is a wonderful tool. Please use it.

Final note: Cyril died after I had completed my initial draft of this chapter. I have spoken to Kathleen a few times since, and the happy memory of what music brought him in his last months, the effect it had on him and indeed the pleasure it gave her to see it, is one that will always be with her. It made her think about his funeral and what to have played. She has chosen the song 'Bring Me Sunshine'.

* * *

For additional information about implementing Namaste Care, a team at Worcester University are developing useful tools arising from their research into Namaste Care in care homes. For example: www.worcester. ac.uk/documents/Guidance-for-Namaste-Care-Workers-V3-updated.pdf Their film, *Seeing is Believing*, is a great summary of Namaste Care: www. youtube.com/watch?v=2kSnvJxScUM.

There are also some films available about Namaste Care on Joyce Simard's website: https://namastecare.com/namaste-care-videos.

11

ENCOURAGING MOVEMENT AND EXERCISE ACTIVITIES AS DEMENTIA PROGRESSES

Magda Pasak, Physiotherapist, St Cuthbert's Hospice, Durham

The old saying of 'use it or lose it' is true for everyone when it comes to our activity levels and it is never too late to start exercising. With a progressive condition like dementia, we can't prevent physical deterioration but we can certainly continue movement for as long as possible to help maintain a good quality of life and make personal care tasks as easy as possible.

When thinking about encouraging a person to exercise, it is important to choose activities that are suitable for them and that they find enjoyable. Exercise can be done individually, with one-to-one supervision or in a small group. Some people may like to try a few different activities to see what suits them best.

People in the different stages of dementia may experience new difficulties in sports and other physical activities they have previously always enjoyed. However, they can be encouraged to continue these activities where possible. Even when nursing and other associated staff or family understand the need for exercise, they may 'refer for physiotherapy' rather than using everyday opportunities to promote movement. However, it is not appropriate just to wait for intermittent physiotherapy input or assume that this will be adequate for care. Walking the patient to the dining table rather than serving a meal at the bedside or helping the patient to make their way to the bathroom rather than putting them in a wheelchair (to save time or thinking it is 'safer') are ways of reducing the complications that give rise to increased dependency. Walking, gardening, dancing and housework are also good forms of everyday physical activity.

The following are ways in which being less mobile can have an effect on the body:

- Weight gain.
- Loss of appetite and possibly weight loss.
- Constipation.
- Fluid build-up in parts of the body such as the feet and legs.
- Skin sensitivity or pressure ulcers due to sitting or lying in the same position for long periods of time.
- Loss of muscle strength, which can mean activities become more difficult or tiring.
- Joint stiffness and a decrease in flexibility.
- Low mood and anxiety.
- Loss in muscle strength and mass, less mobile and stiffer joints, as well as gait changes affect a person's balance and may significantly compromise their mobility.
- Bone density begins to decline after the age of 40, but this loss accelerates around the age of 50. As a result of this bone loss, older people are more prone to fractures. Exercises may help to reduce the risk of bone loss and osteoporosis. Weight-bearing exercises, in particular, help to keep bones healthy and strong.
- Increased risk of various diseases, including cardiovascular disease and stroke.

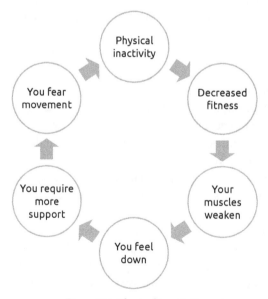

Figure 11.1: Physical inactivity cycle

To avoid this cycle, everyday tasks in daily living can be used to encourage movement and exercise. However, here are some further suggestions for facilitated movement.

CHAIR-BASED EXERCISES

People with dementia can benefit from a regular programme of seated exercise sessions at home or with a group at a local class. It is often a good idea to see these exercises demonstrated at least once by an instructor/physiotherapist or on a video. These exercises are aimed at building or maintaining muscle strength and balance and are less strenuous than exercises in a standing position. They can be part of a developing programme, with the number of repetitions of each exercise increased over time.

The following points should be considered to enable the best outcome for the person with dementia:

- Approach the person from the front making good eye contact at their level.
- Ensure they are addressed with their preferred name.
- Use short instructions and be courteous.
- Keep hand movements open and welcoming, reducing the risk of misinterpretation.
- Do not hurry the person.
- Use a positive tone of voice and have a friendly smile.
- Keep things simple, with one command at a time.
- Break the task down into steps.
- Make the task relevant to the person (e.g. 'Let's go and look out of the window' or 'Let's fold some clothes').

Examples of seated exercises (great with some lively music) are:

- marching on the spot
- turning the upper body from side to side
- raising the heels and toes
- raising the arms towards the ceiling
- raising the opposite arm and leg
- bending the legs
- clapping under the legs
- bicycling the legs and arms (pedal exercises)
- making circles with the arms
- practising moving from sitting to standing.

OTHER FORMS OF EXERCISE
Walking
Walking suits all abilities. It is free, does not need specialist equipment and can be done anywhere. The distance and time spent walking can be varied to suit fitness levels. Some local leisure centres and other organizations arrange group walks of various lengths, supported by a walk leader, so walking can be a social activity as well.

Dancing
Dance exercise is an aerobic activity that burns calories, works the heart muscles and is appropriate for any age and level of fitness since it can also be done in a seated position. Dance requires constant movement at your own pace, which elevates the heart rate to pump oxygen faster through your blood. It can increase strength and flexibility, help with staying steady and agile, and reduce stress. It can also be a very social activity and an enjoyable way to participate in exercise.

Dance can take place in a variety of ways and settings, including dancing at home using the person's favourite music, dancing as a couple or in a group (e.g. tea dances), chair dancing and improvised movement involving ribbons, balloons or balls.

Dance therapy encourages seniors to move in different directions from everyday movement. This helps improve overall balance, stamina and walking speed. There are a wide variety of dance exercise programmes for all ages and skill levels, but many people are afraid to try it, thinking you have to know how to dance prior to taking a class. Most dance exercise classes require no formal training and are taught in a way that anyone can do it.

Tai chi
This ancient Chinese martial art involves breathing, movement, awareness, exercises and meditation. Benefits include: improved quality of movement, balance and co-ordination; reduction in anxiety, depression and stress; and improved concentration. The slow, repeated purposeful movements conducted with a calm and clear state of mind make you more aware of how you move, while improving flexibility and wellbeing. Tai chi can be performed as a seated exercise or standing up, depending on the person's mobility. The classes usually take place in local gyms, hospices and day services.

Using everyday tasks

You can use different household items to make the exercises harder or more interesting. For example:

- Water bottles and soup cans can be used for a lightweight arm workout.
- A towel or a sweatshirt can be pulled taut between the hands to use as a resistance band.
- If you want to be more creative, you can use music and dress according to a particular time period (e.g. wear a 1950s dress and spray the person's favourite scent in the room to remind them of that time).
- Playdoh, sand or a bag of rice can be used to exercise the hands and fingers. This will keep the joints flexible and help with everyday tasks such as writing, getting dressed, grasping or picking up objects. It also provides a nice sensation!
- The person can grab and release handfuls of sand or rice while turning and twisting their hands at the wrist to work the muscles in the hands and fingers.

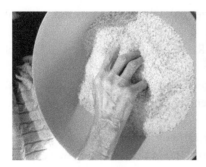 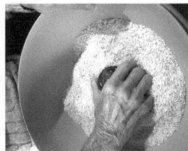

The exercises and activities will not make hand pain and stiffness go away, but stretching helps to get more blood flowing to the hands, increase movement and manage tightness. The sense of touch can be developed by feeling and manipulating objects.

The benefits of sand/rice play include:

- maintenance of fine motor skills
- eye and hand co-ordination – watching and doing and co-ordinating these actions
- promoting creativity and imagination and developing stories
- sensory stimulation – exploring with the sense of touch.

Passive movement

Range of motion (ROM) is the term that is used to describe the amount of movement you have in each joint. Every joint in the body has a 'normal' ROM. Joints maintain their normal ROM by being moved. It is therefore very important to move your joints every day. Stiff joints can cause pain and make it hard for you to do normal daily activities or get dressed easily. ROM exercises preserve flexibility and mobility of the joints on which they are performed. They reduce stiffness and can prevent, or at least slow down, the freezing of joints as dementia symptoms progress. They also help to maintain good circulation.

The joints of immobile patients should be exercised on a regular basis using movements carried out for them by a carer to prevent contracture. Each joint requires being exercised through the ROM, and each movement should be repeated a minimum of three times and preferably five times on each joint. Avoid over-exerting the patient and do not continue exercises to the point where the person develops fatigue.

Here are a few practical tips:

- Move the person's arm/leg very slowly and just to the point of resistance.
- Never cause the person pain. Remind the person to let you know if they feel any pain.
- Watch the person's facial expressions (e.g. grimaces/flinching eyes) while doing exercises – sudden changes in facial expression could indicate pain.
- Always support the person's arm/leg using both hands.
- If you notice any spasms or spasticity in the arm being moved, hold the limb firmly without moving it until the spasm settles.
- Do not try to force the person's joint further than it wants to go.
- If you are in any doubt about how far the person's joint will go, underestimate and stay on the side of caution. Ask a physiotherapist or other healthcare professional about the person's full ROM.

The following are some suggested passive movements to try.

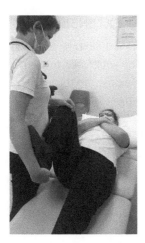

HIP AND KNEE FLEXION

Place one hand on top of the person's knee and cup their foot with your other hand. Raise the person's leg, allowing the hip and knee to bend. Gently push their leg towards their chest. (Their other leg should stay flat on the bed.) Repeat with the other leg.

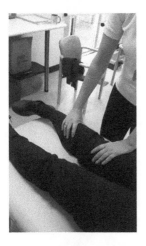

HIP ROTATION

Keeping the person's legs flat on the bed, hold one of their legs above and below the knee, gently rotating the leg inwards and then outwards, monitoring for any resistance. Repeat with the other leg.

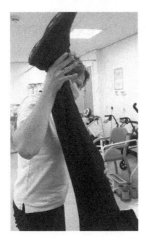

HAMSTRING STRETCH

Place one hand above the person's knee and the other underneath their ankle. Keeping their knee straight, slowly raise their leg. (The other leg should stay flat on the bed.) Repeat with the other leg.

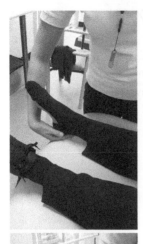

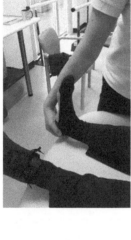

ANKLE FLEXION AND EXTENSION

With the person's leg straight, hold their heel and rest the ball of their foot on your forearm. Gently pull on their heel and apply pressure through the forearm to flex the foot upwards. Then reversing this movement, gently encourage the toes to extend downwards. This exercise encourages ankle flexibility and provides a stretch through the foot. Repeat on the other foot.

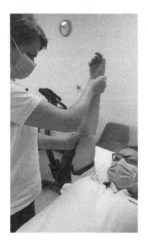

SHOULDER FLEXION AND EXTENSION

Hold the person's wrist with one hand. With the other hand, grasp their elbow joint to stabilize it. Turn their palm inwards, facing the body, and keep their elbow relatively straight. Move their arm from the side of their body over their head. Repeat with the other shoulder.

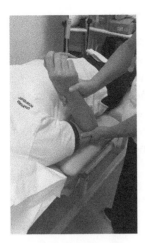

ELBOW FLEXION AND EXTENSION

This can be done with the person in a sitting or lying position. Hold the person's wrist with one hand and place your other hand under their elbow joint. Bend their arm at the elbow joint, up towards the body. The stretch is essentially like a biceps curl (with the hand cupped around the elbow and the thumb pointing out/away from the body). Repeat with the other arm.

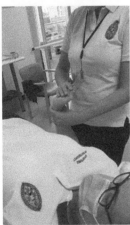

WRIST FLEXION AND EXTENSION

This can be done with the person in a sitting or lying position. Gently bend their wrist towards the inside of the arm (flexion) and then bend the wrist towards the back of the arm (extension). Repeat with the other wrist.

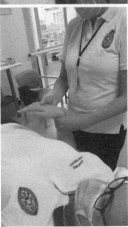

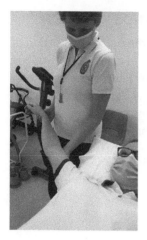

SHOULDER ABDUCTION

Only do this with the person lying down. Keep the person's arm straight, their wrist neutral and their elbow straight with their thumb up (pointing towards the ceiling). The person's arm is gently and smoothly moved in an arc from their side, up towards their ear or as far as it will reach without forcing it. Repeat with the other arm.

CONCLUSION

Carers want to do the best they can for those they are caring for and can be empowered to really make a difference in the level of daily exercise that the person living with dementia experiences. The benefits of exercise to the physical and mental health of the person can positively enhance their quality of life right up until the end of life. The carer will also benefit from an increase in the person's exercise levels, given that it is so important that they too take good care of themselves.

Section 3

SENSORY STORIES AND ACTIVITIES

IN THE ROSE GARDEN

The smell of roses always reminds me of my lovely Grandma. She liberally doused all of the soft toys, dolls and embroidered cushions that she made in rose essential oil. The smell immediately transports me back to my 'Nana' – cuddles by the fire and being loved. I also have fond memories of family trips with my parents to Wynyard Hall rose garden in the Tees Valley and admiring the beautiful colours and smells. There is something tranquil and serene about a rose garden.

Roses tend to flower in the summer, so we can use this special flower to orientate a person living with dementia to that time of year and the season. Many people will have memories of family members taking great pride in their roses, and when I carry out life story work, it is often a favourite flower.

Ideas for sensory resources

- Roses (with thorns removed) to touch, and to display in a vase.
- A realistic butterfly.
- Rose-scented room spritz.
- Rose perfume or body spray.
- Rose-scented hand cream or massage oil.
- A bowl containing cold water for people to put their hands in.
- Rose water and cotton wool to cleanse and refresh the face.
- Hairbrush to brush hair and a rose hair accessory.
- Rose-flavoured tea, Turkish delight, rose-scented cocktail (or mocktail).
- Nature-based relaxing music, including bird song and running water if possible.

To read aloud:

'In the Rose Garden'

Roses in bloom, it must be June.

A delicate, floral scent sweetens the summer air.

I open the garden gate, which creaks on old, worn hinges.

The rose garden is peaceful but not silent. Bird song and the buzz of bees provide Nature's melody.

Somewhere in the distance, gentle music is playing and it relaxes me.

As I walk along the path, I pause to touch the soft, velvet blooms.

A butterfly dances in the air and then comes to rest on a rose, before flitting off again, over the garden wall.

I find the garden seat and sit, taking a deep, relaxing breath, and dipping my hand into the little stream of water flowing from the fountain.

I feel relaxed and safe, surrounded by all types of roses – tea roses, floribundas, a pale-pink damascene.

I rest here, opening up a secret little parcel of tissue paper to reveal a sweet treat, all for me.

I always find a little piece of heaven, here in the rose garden. *Why don't you join me?*

* If ending the second read-through, say: *'I'm so happy you joined me.'*

CITY LIFE

Naturally, someone who spent their life living or working in the city will have very different memories and sensory profiles compared to someone who lived in a rural setting. Some people will feel right at home in the hustle and bustle of the city and so we can attempt to honour that with this story.

Ideas for sensory resources

- Traffic sounds; music from films associated with the city.
- A newspaper the person has always liked to read.
- Smell of fresh coffee.
- Favourite hot beverage to drink and a favourite snack to eat.
- Neon lights and advertising signs.
- If the person has worked in the city, any items related to work, such as a briefcase.
- Vibrant, zesty massage oils, such as bergamot, sweet orange, black pepper.

To read aloud:

'City Life'
Busy, busy, busy in the city.
I walk along the pavement [or 'sidewalk'/'path'] towards my favourite coffee
    stop.
I have to dodge the people rushing off to work.
Newspaper sellers call, so I stop to buy one.
Sounds of cars and buses fill the morning air.
I love the buzz and life of the city.
The lights and advertising signs fill my vision with colour.
Then I reach my destination and the smell of coffee invites me in.
I order my usual – they know me well.
I can rest for a while in this cosy, cosmopolitan oasis and watch the world
    go by.

SPRINGTIME

After the dark days of Winter, people look forward to the change of the season and the lightening of the days as Spring approaches. There's a change in the air, isn't there? People comment on it. There's a definite feeling of the sap rising and the birds getting busy with their nests. The lightness of this season is uplifting and we can convey this by our choice of music, scents and surroundings.

Ideas for sensory resources

- Bulbs and spring flowers (e.g. the smell of freesia placed in a vase on a fresh white, lace tablecloth.
- Tree branches in bud.
- Items and foods associated with Spring festivals (e.g. Easter).
- An uplifting, floral massage oil blend.
- Relaxing music which includes bird song.
- Drinks and food which are culturally associated with Spring (e.g. Easter eggs, spiced cake and other sweet treats).
- Movement activity using chiffon, pastel-coloured scarves.
- Items for a craft activity (e.g. painted eggs).

To read aloud:

'Springtime'
Spring is in the air! Can you feel it?
Everywhere birds are busy finding sticks to build their nests.
It's wonderful to sit and watch them hard at work.
The bulbs are pushing up into the light to bring us their Spring blooms.
They peep at us, new and green from the soil, promising new growth with the new season.
Trees are bursting into bud with new life too.
The days are lightening and the skies are brightening.
Even a Spring shower can't dampen our mood when Spring has sprung.
So, let's shake off the Winter blues and enjoy the new season.

RAINY DAY

I remember once in Florida being caught in the rain and taking shelter on a long porch which had a row of rocking chairs. It was so peaceful sitting under cover, watching the rain. Lots of people will comment on the soothing sound of rain on a tent, caravan or car. This story attempts to create that cosy feeling of watching the rain from a warm, dry, safe place.

Ideas for sensory resources

- Rainmaker or rattle.
- Music related to rain – soothing nature music, including rain, popular songs on the rain theme, such as 'Singin' in the Rain' or 'Raindrops Keep Fallin' on my Head'.
- Plants and a small watering can. (You can water the plants.)
- Bowl of cold water, maybe with leaves or petals floating in it, for the person to put their hands in.
- An umbrella.
- A fresh, herbal scent such as rosemary, pine, cedar or thyme.
- Massage oil.
- Hot chocolate and biscuits.

To read aloud:

'Rainy Day'
It's a day to stay indoors alright!
Dark skies and the pitter-patter of rain on the window pane.
I love the sound it makes. I find it soothing, don't you?
'It's good for the garden,' all the gardeners will be saying. 'Those plants need some water.'
A day for staying inside, warm and dry, listening to music and relaxing.
How about a hot chocolate and some biscuits for a treat, as we stay cosy and warm?
Outside might be wet and cold, but we're safe and peaceful here.
Our little haven, away from the storm.

SCHOOL DAYS

We look back on school days with wistful reminiscence. There were always colourful characters among the teachers and classmates who stood out for all the wrong reasons, or maybe because they were our friends. But either way, school days were our formative years and can bring back a feeling of pleasure and youth. Take the precaution of finding out whether a person had a particularly traumatic time at school, through bullying or because they struggled in lessons; if that is the case, it may not be useful to use this themed activity and story.

Ideas for sensory resources

- Chalk and a small blackboard.
- Adult colouring books.
- Pens, pencils, wooden ruler.
- Exercise books; reference books to look at.
- Sounds the person may associate with school (e.g. a bell).
- Games and toys associated with the school yard (e.g. ball, skipping rope).
- Snacks and drinks associated with school (e.g. juice or milk in a carton, tuck shop sweets in a paper bag).

To read aloud:

'School Days'
Whether we liked it or not, we had to go to school!
Lined up in rows inside the classroom, listening to the teacher.
The click and scrape of chalk on the blackboard, then copying into our
    exercise books.
The smell of the wooden desks and maybe the school dinners being made.
When the bell rang for end of lesson, we gleefully spilled outside to play.
Chatter and squeals as games were played, friendships made and lost.
Then the bell rings again and we line up to traipse back inside.
Cramming our heads (or trying to) with more facts and figures.
We all had our favourite lessons and our favourite teacher.
We wished those days away, those school days, but now they are fond
    memories of the young person we were.

WASH DAY

Families often used to, and some still do, keep to the same day of the week as 'wash day'. It was part of the familiar weekly rhythms of the household, and much pride was taken in the washing, drying, starching and ironing involved. People will frequently say that they enjoyed getting into bed when the sheets were clean on the bed – the cool, fresh experience of clean bed linen is one of those small sensory joys in life for some people. When reminiscing, the person living with dementia may be able to tell you about their memories of the soap powder their mother used, or the twin tub their granny had. Some people even remember the days of the poss tub and mangle!

Note: I am very aware of the gender stereotype contained in this story but make no apologies as it reflects the reality of what the people we support will describe from their childhood. If you know that their circumstances were different, for example if they lived with their grandma or just their father, you could swap 'mother' with whoever is appropriate.

Ideas for sensory resources

- Laundry basket, pegs; rig up a washing line.
- Clothes, small towels to hang up to dry.
- Laundry brush.
- Laundry soap (an old-style brand if possible).
- Old-fashioned wash tub.
- Freshly laundered towels to fold.
- Tea and biscuits.

To read aloud:

'Wash Day'
Monday, so it must be wash day!
'It's a good drying day,' says mother, gathering up the dirty clothes in a
    big pile.
The kitchen is soon filled with the sounds and smell of laundry being
    scrubbed and washed and rinsed.
Sheets are hung out and are soon dancing in neat rows in the breeze.
I can tell mother gets satisfaction from seeing things clean and tidy.
I have to wash my hands before I help her fold the towels – she doesn't
    want them getting grubby when they've just been washed.
Once all the jobs are done, I sit with her on the back step and we have tea
    and biscuits.
'Another good job done,' mother will say with a nod, 'until you lot make
    more work for me.'

A TROPICAL EVENING

Many life stories I hear involve precious memories of special foreign holidays to the likes of the Caribbean, Thailand, Hawaii, India or Africa. These may be holidays which people have saved hard for; maybe they were to celebrate an anniversary or retirement and so have additional fond memories attached. If we can evoke a feeling of a mellow, tropical evening – no hurry and with exotic smells, sounds and tastes – well, that's got to have us feeling relaxed and happy, right?

Ideas for sensory resources

- Subdued lighting (and it should be *evening*).
- Appropriate music (e.g. Caribbean, mellow reggae/saxophone, Indian sitar), ideally with the sound of gentle waves. (Encourage dancing to the music.)
- Tropical fruit to taste.
- Fruit juice rum cocktails/mocktails.
- Coconut, mango or other suitable tropical-scented hand cream, or massage oil with an exotic scent such as ylang ylang or patchouli. (Songbird do a massage wax called 'Pacific Nights', for example.)
- Grass skirts and flower garlands.
- Hawaiian shirts to wear.
- A bowl of warm water with flower petals floating in it, for the person to dip their hands into.

To read aloud:

'A Tropical Evening'
Sundown, by a tropical sea, is where I want to be!
Mellow music soaks through me like sweet molasses, and all my stress floats away on a warm ocean breeze.
I sway to the beat, I just can't help it. My body just wants to dance.
There's nothing to do and nowhere to be, other than relaxing right here, in this special moment.
I want to dip my toes in those gentle, lapping waves. I've got all the time in the world.
Then I'll sit back and enjoy the exotic tastes of fruit and rum, all having a party on my tongue.
A tropical evening, surrounded by lush green palms, lulls my senses, soothes my soul.
It's my kind of bliss.

A DESERT OASIS

Thinking about creating a diverse range of sensory experiences, I wondered about the rich sensory experiences that must be offered by a desert oasis. I've never been to one, and many of the people we support probably won't have been to one either. But they will have watched films and have an archetypal sense of this environment, which it may be nice to offer to them through this sensory story.

Ideas for sensory resources

- Moroccan, Egyptian or Middle-Eastern music.
- Chiffon scarves, belly dancing coin belts, rich silk fabrics, Hamman-style fringed towels.
- Musical instruments (e.g. rattles, tambourine, finger cymbals and small drums).
- Exotic fruits (e.g. figs, dates, pomegranate juice, sweet tea and other foods related to desert areas).
- Musky smells (e.g. diluted frankincense, myrrh, patchouli oil, or use incense sticks).
- A bowl or paddling pool of lukewarm water filled with petals and scented oils for the person to dip their hands into or paddle in.
- Electric fan to create a breeze.
- A heater, if needed, to raise the room temperature.
- Pictures of a desert oasis, maybe a nature film or a classic film featuring an oasis.

To read aloud:

'A Desert Oasis'
For travellers in the desert, an oasis really is a heavenly sight.
A little haven of lush green awaits you, surrounding a beautiful pool of
    fresh, spring water.
Exotic music drifts on the breeze, as the palm trees rustle gently, as if
    they're dancing.
And you want to dance too. Don't be shy.
Let your body sway and shimmy to the music like those belly dancers do.
Our bodies were made to move, and we love to dance, don't we?
Move to the rhythm, shake to the beat.
Now, it's time to rest.
Breathe in the musky scents and enjoy this place of comfort and safety.
Put your weary feet into the refreshing water and relax.
We've made an oasis of calm to make you smile and soothe your soul.

POET'S CORNER

There's something about the rhythm of poetry which people living with dementia seem to find very soothing. They may well have had favourite poets and poems or they may not have read much poetry at all, but there is an innate appreciation of poetry which seems to endure for people living with dementia. The repetition of pattern and routine does appear to assist a person living with dementia in everyday life, and so maybe a poem is a representation of this.

Ideas for sensory resources

- Poetry books, old books to handle.
- Classical music or mellow jazz.
- Candles.
- Lemongrass massage oil (helps to make the person feel relaxed and alert).
- Flame playing on TV screen.
- Cosy blankets and cushions.
- Hot drink and biscuits.

To read aloud:

'Poet's Corner'
Poems paint the colours of the world in words.
The beauty of poetry is timeless and touches our hearts.
Happy and sad, passionate and poignant, we listen to the words weaved together by the poet.
Let's get ourselves cosy and warm, and spend some time enjoying some verse.
We can hear from the great poets, who speak to us in rhyme and prose.
We can drift away on a lazy afternoon, letting the words sink into our souls.
Let's open the book and browse.
What poem shall we choose, just for you?

BY THE SEA

A frequent feature in life stories are memories of day trips to the beach, or holidays by the sea. Childhood carefree days of sandcastles, kite flying, ice cream and picnics with sand between our toes and also in the sandwiches! Seagulls, rock pools, exploring, paddling or swimming. All happy memories we can attempt to recreate.

Ideas for sensory resources

- Music associated with the seaside, or a calming soundscape including waves.
- Pebbles, shells (check for sharp edges), dried seaweed, driftwood.
- A sand tray filled with sand, and some small buckets and spades.
- A fan to create a small breeze.
- A bowl of water or paddling pool for paddling.
- A beach towel to dry feet on.
- A knotted handkerchief.
- Hand cream or body lotion containing seaweed, or with a sea-related theme/smell.
- Ice cream, candy floss, chips (fries) in cones.

To read aloud:

'By the Sea'
'Oh, I do like to be beside the seaside,' or so the old song goes!
But it's true isn't it? A day by the sea is always a happy day.
I could sit for hours letting sand run through my fingers, the sea breeze on my face.
I couldn't help myself, I always had to pick up things that caught my eye.
Maybe a pretty pebble, a shell, or some other little treasure washed up on the shore.
I loved to paddle, the cool water lapping at my ankles and the sand moving beneath my feet.
And oh, how I used to laugh at Grandad in his deck chair, with his knotted hankie on his bald head to keep the sun off!
There were always treats too – it was a treat sort of a day.
Ice cream cones, with sand between your toes, and the sound of the waves on the shore.
Can you think of anything better than a day at the seaside to boost your spirits?

PICNIC IN THE MEADOW

Sitting on a picnic rug amongst the tall grass and the wildflowers of a summer meadow was the inspiration for this little story. Long, lazy summer afternoons spent cloud watching, listening to the birds and making daisy chains come to mind. And of course, everyone loves a picnic. Let's share this feeling.

Ideas for sensory resources

- Picnic rug/blanket.
- Old-style picnic basket filled with a picnic lunch, a flask for hot drinks or a jug of homemade lemonade.
- Pots of tall grasses or an area in the garden which has been allowed to grow wild with meadow flowers and tall grass.
- A portable old-style radio.
- Hats and a garden parasol.
- A light massage oil containing some drops of an appropriate essential oil (e.g. chamomile).

To read aloud:

'Picnic in the Meadow'
What a gorgeous day for a picnic!
Trailing our hands through the long grass; here we've found the perfect spot.
Delicate wildflowers nod their heads as a light breeze dances over the meadow.
The sweet scent of flowers and the earthy smell of grass fill the air.
Birds sing to us from a nearby tree, and little white fluffy clouds drift lazily across a blue, sunny sky.
We need hats and a parasol to give us some shade from the bright summer sun.
Let's spread out our picnic blanket and lay out our picnic.
Then we'll switch on the radio while we tuck into our lunch.
There's nowhere to go and nothing to do.
So, sit back and relax on a lazy, summer afternoon.

IN THE SHADE OF THE TREE

When you sit underneath a tree, you can feel the atmosphere change. It's like a little sacred space where time slows and we can connect with nature. If there is a tree to take people to sit under, that would be wonderful; but if not, try the various sensory resources to link with the idea of tree and wisdom and being at peace with a life lived.

Ideas for sensory resources

- Bark, leaves, branches, pine cones, acorns, logs, etc. to touch.
- A nature film/screensaver with soundscape.
- Face cream and hand cream.
- A hand-held mirror.
- Seedlings to plant in compost or water.
- Essential oils (e.g. cedarwood atlas, pine or similar).
- Food treats related to trees (e.g. maple syrup, birch bark drinks, cakes including nuts [being aware of allergies and swallowing difficulties]).
- You could encourage movement during the story, such as stretching arms up to the sky and down to the ground.

To read aloud:

'In the Shade of the Tree'
I love to sit in the dappled shade of my favourite big old tree.
Branches stretch a protective canopy above, up to the sky, and roots reach
    deep down into the earth.
Leaves rustle and dance in the breeze, while time seems to slow...right...
    down.
This wise old tree must have seen many people come and go; just think of it.
Running my fingers over the gnarled, rough bark, I think of my own skin
    which is weathered and wrinkled with the smiles and frowns of life.
Those lines on my face are the marks of experience in my elder years.
I nod to myself with a knowing smile.
I wear a wealth of life lived, there on my face, just like this wise old tree.

FRESHLY BAKED BREAD

There are many things that express our country, culture and individual preferences, and bread is one of them. Whether it is Middle-Eastern flatbread, Greek pitta, Indian chapati, German pumpernickel, Irish soda bread or my beloved North East English stottie, love of bread is pretty universal (unless you are gluten intolerant!).

Ideas for sensory resources

- Freshly baked bread which is still warm.
- Various accompaniments – butter, jam, cheese, olive oil, etc., according to local traditions and personal preferences.
- Baker's hat, apron, oven gloves, stalks of wheat.
- Old photographs of baker's shops.
- Mood lamp with warm colours of gold and orange.
- Music, maybe associated with bread advertising or harvest.
- Items for possible activity: salt dough (large mixing bowl, 2 cups flour, 1 cup salt, ¾ cup water) to knead, shape and bake at 180°C.

To read aloud:

'Freshly Baked Bread'
There isn't anything quite like the delicious smell of freshly baked bread.
The baker starts his day bright and early, making all kinds of delights.
Kneading, shaping, proving, baking. A wizard with dough!
He displays the loaves proudly in his shop, ready for us to take home and try.
What is your favourite way to enjoy bread?
I like mine with lashings of fresh butter and jam. What about you?
No street is complete without a good baker's shop.
Now, let's relax and break some bread together.

AUTUMN REFLECTIONS

I always think of Autumn as a time for quiet reflection. There's a definite change in the air as the days cool and trees change colour. People often comment on this, don't they? It's a time of harvest and preparing for Winter and a time to say goodbye to Summer. For many people, as children, Autumn meant a return to school or college after the summer break. All these associations are written into our memory and can be evoked as the season changes. Cosiness, quiet time and comfort are the themes.

Ideas for sensory resources

- Crisp, dried leaves, acorns, pine cones, etc. in a box.
- Cosy knitted blankets.
- Woody or musky smells; smell of an open fire.
- A screensaver film on the TV of an open fire.
- Mellow, relaxing music.
- Maybe a nature film about Autumn.
- Marshmallows which can perhaps be toasted on behalf of the person for safety.
- Hot chocolate to drink.

To read aloud:

'Autumn Reflections'
Mother Nature must surely be an artist, with the trees as her canvas.
This time of year, she touches the leaves with Autumn shades of red, orange, gold and brown, so that we know that it is time to let go of Summer.
We'll be thankful for the harvest; apples and pears are ripe and ready.
The smell of garden fires drifts in the air, as the days cool and darken.
It's a cosy time of blankets and toasted marshmallows and hot chocolate.
We might remember the days we returned to school after the summer break. That 'new term' feeling that Autumn brings.
But most of all, it's a time to pause and reflect on the changing of the seasons and the turning of the year once more.
The tides of life, and the rhythm of the year, painted in the colours of Autumn.

WINTER'S STARK BEAUTY

Winter is my favourite season, but I know that is not true for everyone. I love the cold and getting wrapped up warm against the chill. I have known Namaste Care volunteers take boxes full of snow into the house for people living with dementia to touch – that certainly is a direct way to bring the outdoors inside! Winter will mean many different things for different people. Maybe there are festivals that are meaningful too, like Diwali, Thanksgiving or Christmas. For me, in Northern Europe, it is cold and trees have lost their leaves, bringing a stark beauty to the landscape, but I would urge you to shape a story of your own if this does not fit your particular type of Winter.

Ideas for sensory resources

- Paper snowflakes.
- Crushed ice in a bowl.
- Sprigs of evergreen foliage such as fir tree branches.
- Hats, scarves and gloves to wear.
- Nature film of snowy landscapes.
- A misting diffuser with a blue mood lamp colour, or candle.
- Warm, spiced smells (e.g. orange cinnamon candles and oil blends).
- Toasted muffins, roast chestnuts, warm spiced drinks (maybe with a nip of whisky) and any other appropriate seasonal food and drink.
- Relaxing music.

To read aloud:

'Winter's Stark Beauty'

The trees have lost their Autumn leaves and now seem to be sleeping.

The world seems painted in shades of white and grey, as frost makes patterns on the window panes.

Snowflakes flutter from a heavy sky, silent and beautiful.

A chill wind blows in from the North, and everyone is wrapping up warm against the cold.

Stamping feet and rubbing hands, our breath making little clouds as we speak.

But inside, cuddled up cosy and warm, we can watch Winter's stark beauty and smile.

A time to rest and enjoy good company, seasonal food and drinks that cheer our soul.

Winter festivals with fairy lights and twinkling candles fill the darkest days.

Evergreen branches and sprigs remind us that life goes on and the light will return.

The gentle, dormant time of Winter hibernation isn't so bad after all.

A MOUNTAIN STREAM

Thinking about capturing special moments took me to a family day in the Welsh mountains on a warm summer day, clambering over rocks with my children and cooling off with our feet in the icy cold stream. We had a picnic and it was so relaxing. I'm guessing many people might have memories like this, whether it in mountains in your own country or when you have travelled abroad. I also remember a mountain stream in the Alps with my parents as a child, eating apple strudel at a café by the stream on a glorious blue-sky day. So, let's try to capture some of that.

Ideas for sensory resources

- A bowl of cold water with rocks and pebbles in the bottom for dipping hands into, and a larger bowl or paddling pool of cold water to put feet into.
- Pine essential oil in a room spray or diffuser.
- Songbird massage wax – 'Mountain Forest' blend or similar, or a massage oil containing a pine or cedar essential oil.
- Nature sounds, including the sound of a stream (sound machine or music).
- Food associated with mountains that the person would recognize (e.g. for the Alps, apple strudel, goats cheese, Swiss chocolate; for the English Lake District, Kendal mint cake or Grasmere gingerbread, etc.).
- General picnic foods.

To read aloud:

'A Mountain Stream'
I remember a happy day spent by a mountain stream.
The sound of water dancing and gurgling over rocks is so soothing.
The smell of pine trees drifting on the fresh mountain breeze makes me
    take a deep breath in and sigh.
I reach into the icy cold water of the stream, searching for the beautiful
    pebbles made smooth by the water and the passing of the years.
Then it's off with socks and shoes to cool off with my feet dangling in the
    refreshing water.
It's a carefree feeling, as time seems to stand still.
Little white clouds drift lazily gently across a blue sky as I feel all my stress
    wash away in this gentle mountain stream.
Time for a picnic and a drink, wishing this special moment could last forever.

DRUM BEAT

There is something primal and comforting about the sound of a drum beat. Maybe it is the first sound we hear – the regular, reassuring beat of our mother's heartbeat in the womb. Using a drum can be energetic, or relaxing and hypnotic, depending on the volume, the type of drum and the pace. If the person living with dementia wants to participate, you can offer them a drum stick, beater or a bongo type drum to pat. Rattles are also useful as they are light and easy to handle and keep a beat with.

Ideas for sensory resources

- Various types of drums, beaters and rattles.
- Music which features different distinct drum beats, such as native American music, military bands, African tribal music.
- Smells which link to the wood the drums are made of (e.g. pine or cedarwood essential oils).
- Herbal teas and healthy snacks (this is what I associate with drums, but it could be beer and bar snacks).

To read aloud:

'Drum Beat'
Listen to the voice of the drum…
Boom-boom…boom-boom *[on the drum]*
Like a steady heart…beating time
Boom-boom…boom-boom *[on the drum]*
Like ancient feet, beating the earth, dancing
Boom-boom…boom-boom *[on the drum and add in stamping feet]*
I am what I am, says the drum
Boom-boom…boom-boom *[on the drum]*
Let's play…
Boom-boom…boom-boom *[on the drum]*

An alternative drum option is to read aloud in a rhythmic voice:

'Move to the Beat of the Drum'
Listen to the drum…like a heart…beating…
Doum-doum…doum-doum…
That primal, earthy sound, regular and strong…like a pulse of power
Doum-doum…doum-doum…
Find your rhythm and just let go…
Doum-doum…doum-doum…

Your body wants to move to the beat...
Doum-doum...doum-doum...
Why don't you clap your hands and stamp your feet?
Doum-doum...doum-doum
Through all of history...the drum has sounded...beating time...
Doum-doum...doum...
Let's lose our poise and just make some noise...
Doum-doum...doum-doum...

A CAT CALLED 'WHISKY'

Families can feel conflicted about whether the use of realistic toys and dolls is adult-appropriate. Having seen the joyful responses they bring to people living with dementia, however, I would personally say that this judgement of them being childish is us seeing things through our own filters and I would not want to deprive people of an opportunity if it is something that brings comfort. I recently saw the absolute delight on the face of an ex-army man when the very realistic robotic toy cat his family had bought for him miaowed at him for attention. 'There, there' and a gentle pat was his response. This story was written for him.

Ideas for sensory resources

- A realistic cat toy (there are lots now available specifically for people living with dementia).
- Music from *Cats* the musical, or other cat-related music.
- A cat collar with a bell.
- Tea and biscuits (or any other relaxing refreshments).
- Relaxing blend of room spray.
- Films or documentaries about cats (e.g. *The Secret Life of Cats*) available on BBC, Netflix, National Geographic, YouTube.

To read aloud:

'A Cat Called "Whisky"'
She's furry and she's purry and just a little bit sassy.
A cat called Whisky is our very own feline princess.
A tinkle of her bell announces she's arrived, so pay attention to her Royal Highness!
Like cat royalty, she surveys her loyal subjects and decides where to settle down.
With her soft, silky fur and sleek green eyes, we can't help but fall in love with her.
…And she knows it!
She cuddles into us; we can't help but sit back and relax.
She loves to be stroked and adored, of course.
But as she begins to get sleepy and breathe deeper, we also feel all our tension melt away.
So that we breathe a little deeper too, and dream away the day in cat heaven.

MAN'S BEST FRIEND

Joyce Simard has a very adorable dog hand puppet called Bella. A big, furry Old English Sheepdog that nuzzles and cuddles and never fails to raise a smile and a chuckle. If the person living with dementia has owned a dog themselves or one has been part of the family, it can be great to bring in a friendly dog to meet them. It sparks such joy, reaching out and engagement (in the same way that small children so often do). In the absence of a real dog, a realistic toy or puppet would be great. So, this story is in honour of Joyce and Bella.

Ideas for sensory resources

- A real dog, or a realistic toy dog or puppet.
- A ball and toys for the dog; maybe a dog grooming brush.
- A bowl of water for handwashing.
- Herbal-scented hand cream or massage wax.
- Dog-themed music (e.g. 'Hound Dog' and 'How Much Is That Doggie in the Window?').
- Films related to dogs.
- Snacks and drinks.

To read aloud:

'Man's Best Friend'
Who can resist a wagging tail and those big, soulful eyes?
They say man's best friend is his dog, don't they?
Loyal and true, they are a loving and faithful companion.
They never argue or answer back. They never let us down.
Meet this gorgeous bundle of fur and give him some love.
Stroking a dog helps us feel calm and adored.
Playing with our dog cheers us up on the glummest of days.
With a dog in your life, you'll never be lonely or sad.

AS THE SUN GOES DOWN

Many people living with dementia go through a phase of 'sundowning' where they are very unsettled and more disorientated in the evening. Getting into a routine which signals it's time to settle down and bedtime is approaching can help with this disruption to the body clock. This story is therefore designed for *evenings* and could possibly be used every evening to get the person living with dementia into a rhythm and pattern that feels familiar and safe.

Ideas for sensory resources

- Relaxing music.
- An easy-to-read clock.
- A warm, fuzzy blanket.
- Relaxing room spritz (e.g. lavender or chamomile).
- Hot chocolate, chamomile tea or some other drink associated with bedtime.
- Night clothes laid out.
- Subdued, warm-coloured lighting.

To read aloud:

'As the Sun Goes Down'
As the sun goes down, everything becomes slower, quieter.
The birds are settling down into their roosts and mellow evening bird song fills the air.
Folks are getting sleepy now after another busy day…yawn.
We're having a lovely, soothing night-time drink as we prepare for bed.
Lazy music helps us wind down…slow down…there's nothing else to do.
And the sun sinks slowly in the sky, so that evening shadows deepen.
The clock ticks…its regular rhythm telling us that it will soon be time for bed.
Time to rest and lay down our weary head.

STORIES FOR END OF LIFE

TIME TO LET GO

THE BUTTERFLY

ALL THAT I AM

Ideas for sensory resources appropriate for the next three stories

- The person's favourite relaxing music.
- A calming room spritz or diffuser (e.g. diluted lemon balm, chamomile or mandarin).
- Subdued, gentle lighting.
- One of the sacred oils such as frankincense, elemi, rose, sandalwood or patchouli diluted in a rich oil such as rapeseed oil (five drops of essential oil in 10ml carrier oil for anointing the chest, brow and crown of the head at end of life) or use the sacred oil blend suggested in Chapter 5.
- Treasured objects and photographs.
- Soft blankets and cushions.
- Flowers or plants.

To read aloud:

'Time to Let Go'

How do we know when it's time to let go?

When our heart keeps on beating, and our breath keeps on breathing.

But there comes a time when our body is tired.

There's a time, when all the days of our life have played out. Every dance has to end, every song has to play out.

And though it will feel like a step into the unknown, it is actually a step into perfect peace.

Where all the pain will be gone and you can rest.

You can finally lay down life's burden and relax.

And your loved ones will cry to see you go, but tears mean that there has been love.

You will go with their blessing, no need for a heavy heart.

So, I whisper to you…dear, beautiful soul…it is time to finally trust…and let go.

To read aloud:

'The Butterfly'

Inside a warm cocoon the caterpillar slept, underneath an oak leaf, hidden and safe.

Its little body was busy changing, transforming, as it slumbered, cosy and secure.

And finally, one fine day, it wriggled gently free from its tight wrappings.

It paused, getting used to a new feeling. A lighter feeling. A brighter feeling.

And then, oh...oh my...

Gently, carefully it unfurled its new, vibrant, colourful wings.

The world paused for a moment to admire the beauty of this little soul and then it lightly...

Just like that...

With barely any effort...

Beat its tiny wings...took to the air...and flew away.

To read aloud:

'All That I Am'

When I die, as we all surely will, how will I measure, all that I am? All that I have been?

I am a million hugs and kisses, wrapped up in fond memories.

I am losses and tragedies lived through and overcome.

I am school days and holidays, and work days and sick days.

I am tears of sadness and laughter blended with the waves on the shore or the days I was caught in the rain.

My physical body is tired and worn out now, that part of who I am is fading.

But who I am, all that I am, the love and memories people hold for me, the energy by which I lived my life... Well, that cannot die.

Like an ever-burning candle flame, that energy will always shine.

Because I have lived, all that I am, the essence of me, will remain.

My life is etched into the history of the universe.

It will be in the twinkle of the stars for those who care to look up. It will be in the breeze upon a blade of grass for those who pause to reflect. It will be in the garden I tended, the photographs I took, the memories I made with friends and family.

So, though parting may seem painful, please know, that all that I am honours all that you are, and when this happens, there is no parting.

CONCLUSION

As my father's dementia progresses, and we have had to support him through repeated chest infections, falls, a never-ending nosebleed and a broken pelvis, the stress and exhaustion for his main carer, my mother, is clear to see. But it ripples throughout all of the family in various ways, from one crisis to another. We have thought we were going to lose him at least three times now – I joke that he's had two more resurrections than Jesus – and it's draining, it really is.

Faced with this rollercoaster of emotions and constant worry for the safety of the person living with dementia, added to the physical demands of helping them with their personal care and the mental strain, it is easy to understand why carers are happy for the person with dementia to sit quiet and safe in front of the TV. What we have given up on though, if we do this, is the joy of life we can generate. The smiles, the magic moments, that special time spent together actually counteracts the feeling of negativity and 'groundhog day' of caring for someone living with dementia.

Human beings are wired to notice the negative. It's a survival mechanism from our ancient evolutionary past. At the end of the day, we tend to reflect and ruminate on the one or two things that have gone wrong, rather than the many neutral or positive things that have happened that day. We brush over a compliment with hardly a second thought, yet we spend hours in negative self-talk about something someone said to us that we didn't like. As a cave dweller who might have encountered wolves and bears, getting it wrong could mean life and death. Nowadays it is rare for us to experience something quite so dramatically life-threatening!

But the negativity bias robs us of our joy. Dementia feeds the negativity bias, big time. It's a life-limiting condition, so of course it does. But it's time to claim back the joy. When something nice happens… *pause*… notice how it feels, revel in it. Talk to people about it. During a recent 'Potting Shed' men's group, I was struggling to engage one of our group members in the gardening task. He had no interest and appeared to be embarrassed that he was unable to do the task, which in the past would have been simple for him. So, I switched the activity and played table quoits with him. My repeated hopeless failed attempts and his scoring on his very first turn soon turned his frown to a smile and then a laugh. We both had a good time. I not only lifted his mood but also my own. When his wife came to collect him, she commented on how upbeat he was and it lasted for the rest of the day. I reported back to my colleagues about it and enjoyed the feeling that I knew I'd made a difference to that man on that day. Negativity bias counteracted!

We can all do this! It's not clever or technical. The negative is there but let's choose to focus on the positive, the relational and the joyful and we may stand a chance of making this dementia journey a little less bumpy.

As I conclude this book, I hope it can serve in a small way to lighten what can feel like the heavy burden of dementia. We can, with a little effort, re-frame the grief to look much more like a celebration of life.

Namaste

Nicola

Recommended Suppliers

IN THE UK

Base Formula: Range of room spritzes, massage oils and waxes, skincare, essential oils and gels

    www.baseformula.com

Songbird: Range of massage waxes

    www.songbirdnaturals.co.uk

Oshadhi: Excellent quality and range of essential oils and carrier oil

    https://oshadhi.co.uk

Soulmidwives Shop: Offers a selection of the sacred oils, and access to online training

    www.soulmidwivesshop.co.uk

Temple Spa: A small, ethical British company making artisan products inspired by Mediterranean ingredients, including skincare, room sprays, massage oils, candles

    www.templespa.com

Unforgettable: Online shop for products specifically designed to support someone living with dementia

    https://dementia.livebetterwith.com/collections/partner-product

ROMPA: Specialist Sensory Equipment and ideas

    www.rompa.com

IN THE USA
Essential oils
Mountain Rose Herbs

http://mountainroseherbs.com

Young Living

https://youngliving.com

Pompeii Organics

https://pompeiiorganics.com

Sources of Inspiration

IDEAS FOR SHARING MUSIC, NATURE FILMS AND MEMORIES (THERE ARE MANY MORE!)

www.playlistforlife.org.uk

www.watershed.co.uk/studio/projects/music-memory-box

https://remarc.bbcrewind.co.uk

https://youtube.com

Recommended Reading

Alzheimer's Net at www.alzheimers.net/2014-01-23/sensory-stimulation-alzheimers-patients.

Doka, K.J. (2009) 'Disenfranchised grief.' *Bereavement Care* 18(3), 37–39.

Gerhardt, S. (2004) *Why Love Matters: How Affection Shapes a Baby's Brain.* Abingdon: Routledge.

Grace, J. (2018) *Sharing Sensory Stories and Conversations with People with Dementia: A Practical Guide.* London: Jessica Kingsley Publishers.

Griffin, J. and Tyrrell, I. (2003) *Human Givens: A New Approach to Emotional Health and Clear Thinking.* Chalvington: Human Givens Publishers.

Kendall, N. (2019) *Namaste Care for People Living with Advanced Dementia: A Practical Guide for Carers and Professionals.* London: Jessica Kingsley Publishers.

Leighton, R., Oddy, C. and Grace, J. (2016) 'Using sensory stories with individuals with dementia.' *Australian Journal of Dementia Care* 5(6), 17–19.

Lindauer, A. and Harvath, T.A. (2014) 'Pre-death grief in the context of dementia caregiving: A concept analysis.' *Journal of Advanced Nursing* 70(10), 2196–2207. DOI:10.1111/jan.12411.

Matthews, J. and Matthews, C. (2009) *Storyworld: The Storytelling Box.* London: Templar.

Simard, J. (2013) *The End of Life Namaste Care Programme for People with Dementia.* Baltimore, MD: Health Professions Press.

Stacpoole, M., Thompsell, A. and Hockley, J. (2016) *Toolkit for implementing the Namaste Care programme for people with advanced dementia living in care homes.* Available at www.stchristophers.org.uk/wp-content/uploads/2016/03/Namaste-Care-Programme-Toolkit-06.04.2016.pdf, accessed on 2 December 2020.

Warner, F. (2018) *Sacred Oils: Working with 20 Precious Oils to Heal Spirit and Soul.* London: Hay House.

Index

Subheadings in *italics* indicate tables and diagrams